FATIGUE

A Step-by-step Guide to Pausing the Adrenals and Balancing the Cortisol

(Chronic Fatigue Syndrome Cure - Basic Guide for Recovery)

Nelda Neill

Published by Oliver Leish

Nelda Neill

All Rights Reserved

Fatigue: A Step-by-step Guide to Pausing the Adrenals and Balancing the Cortisol (Chronic Fatigue Syndrome Cure - Basic Guide for Recovery)

ISBN 978-1-77485-158-6

All rights reserved. No part of this guide may be reproduced in any form without permission in writing from the publisher except in the case of brief quotations embodied in critical articles or reviews.

Legal & Disclaimer

The information contained in this book is not designed to replace or take the place of any form of medicine or professional medical advice. The information in this book has been provided for educational and entertainment purposes only.

The information contained in this book has been compiled from sources deemed reliable, and it is accurate to the best of the Author's knowledge; however, the Author cannot guarantee its accuracy and validity and cannot be held liable for any errors or omissions. Changes are periodically made to this book. You must consult your doctor or get professional medical advice before using any of the suggested remedies, techniques, or information in this book.

Upon using the information contained in this book, you agree to hold harmless the Author from and against any damages, costs, and expenses, including any legal fees potentially resulting from the application of any of the information provided by this guide. This disclaimer applies to any damages or injury caused by the use and application, whether directly or indirectly, of any advice or information presented, whether for breach of contract, tort, negligence, personal injury, criminal intent, or under any other cause of action.

You agree to accept all risks of using the information presented inside this book. You need to consult a professional medical practitioner in order to ensure you are both able and healthy enough to participate in this program.

Table of Contents

INTRODUCTION 1

CHAPTER 1: THE UNEXPLAINABLE FATIGUE 4

CHAPTER 2: WHAT IS CHRONIC FATIGUE SYNDROME? 11

CHAPTER 3: METABOLISM SIMPLIFIED 25

CHAPTER 4: DIET – WHAT TO EAT TO LOOK AND FEEL GOOD 33

CHAPTER 5: UNDERSTANDING THE STRESSORS IN THE MODERN WORKPLACE 36

CHAPTER 6: GET A SCHEDULE 41

CHAPTER 7: BACK TO BASICS 45

CHAPTER 8: WHAT IS OCCUPATIONAL BURNOUT? 54

CHAPTER 9: INTESTINAL SUPPORT 64

CHAPTER 10: HOW MUCH ENERGY WE NEED DAILY 70

CHAPTER 11: FATIGUE FIGHTING VITAMINS AND HERBS. 73

CHAPTER 12: THE DAY I GOT SICK 84

CHAPTER 13: THE HISTORY OF THE FRUITARIAN DIET ... 119

CHAPTER 14: WHAT AGGRAVATES PAIN? 129

- CHAPTER 15: RELAX 135
- CHAPTER 16: LIVING STRONG WITH HYPOTHYROIDISM 140
- CHAPTER 17: MUSCLE FATIGUE 153
- CHAPTER 18: METHODS OF DEALING WITH CHRONIC STRESS 160
- CHAPTER 19: HAVE YOU HEARD OF FIBROMYALGIA? 167
- CHAPTER 20: LOOKING FORWARD TO THE BENEFITS OF BUSTING FATIGUE 169
- CHAPTER 21: INTERNAL STRESS AND HOW TO DEAL WITH IT 174
- CHAPTER 22: WHY DO YOU NEED TESTOSTERONE? 179
- CONCLUSION 183

Introduction

Tiredness and exhaustion are major players contributing to our overall wellbeing. When we feel tired all the time, then our resources are soon depleted, and our emotions can swing all over the place. There are many elements which contribute to maintaining healthy energy levels, most of which I am sure you are well aware of: getting enough sleep, feeling relaxed, eating a healthy diet with organic fruit and veg on a daily basis, drinking plenty of pure water, exercising, etc. Sometimes energy levels are affected by illness such as hypothyroidism or ME, so if you are suffering from long term low energy, check with your doctor to see if there is a medical reason for your tiredness.

Fatigue is something that strikes many people as they go about their workout program. Whether fatigue hits early on or near the end of your workout, if you're aiming to keep your session as intense as possible, there's no question fatigue is cramping your overall style. With a few smart tips and strategies, you can overcome fatigue.

Are you ready to unlock the secret to a more youthful "you"?

Fighting fatigue to live your best life is something we all seek. However, I must point out one important thing:

Many individuals tend to focus too much on "their fatigue" or the causes of fatigue vs. turning their attention to what actually will allow them to feel great. I want to help shift your attention with exclusive information.

If you are experiencing mornings where you can barely get out of bed, Your feeling tired unmotivated to experience the day ahead of you, your feeling miserable throughout the long days of work, your unable to keep a clear state of mind, or your even forcing yourself to combine work, family care, and personal time all in one never finding satisfaction —

Chapter 1: The Unexplainable Fatigue

Described as a complicated disorder, the Chronic fatigue Syndrome (CFS) is an extreme fatigue which can't be described best by any medical condition. With mental or physical activities, the fatigue may aggravate and rest is not enough to improve the condition. Whilst the main cause of chronic fatigue is unknown, there are various factors and theories such as psychological stress and viral infections associated with this syndrome.

Moreover, variety of medical tests is required to confirm the syndrome's diagnosis and help rule out other possibilities and health risks. The treatment focuses more on the relief of the syndrome rather than curing it entirely. In most cases, the syndrome develops after a certain period of stress or flu-like illness. However, it can still occur to people who are not sick. It can develop quietly and gradually and due to its vagueness, the patient might not notice the problem for weeks or even months. Moreover, the diagnosis in unclear making it difficult to predict what is normal with the syndrome.

Most people with chronic fatigue syndrome feel a long-term tiredness that almost disabled them. They usually experience symptoms such as disturbed sleeping patterns, joint pains, muscular pains, headaches and poor concentration. And because its cause is unknown, there are controversies regarding the real nature of the syndrome. The diagnosis can only be made with the presence of certain symptoms that vary in severity and type.

At the onset of each symptom, patients can experience sudden or gradual occurrence. Fatigue is the main symptom of CFS. The persistent fatigue or tiredness may cause a person to limit his activities in the long run. Normally, this can be feeling both mentally and physically and the fatigue is overwhelming. Even getting a complete rest cannot ease the tiredness. Moreover, it can be aggravated by doing any activity.

Other symptoms include poor concentration and loss of memory, short attention span and short-term memory. Other cognitive difficulties are being disoriented, having difficulties in organizing one's though and planning. Other patients also experience sleeping difficulties. Sleeping becomes un-refreshing for them as they would normally have disrupted sleep patterns, wake up to early or unable to create quality sleep.

Recurring sore throat is also a common sign of chronic fatigue syndrome. It is often accompanied with enlarged lymph nodes in the armpits and neck. Moreover, pain is the most prominent among other symptoms. The patient experiences headaches, muscles and joint pains. The pain doesn't come along with redness and swelling but it transfers from joints. Other cases reported symptoms such as sickness, dizziness and palpitations.

The symptoms' severity can be classified into three;

Mild cases - the patient is still able to fulfill light activities and can take care of himself. He can still go to work but would occasionally take a leave. Moreover, the patient should stop engaging in other social activities and should use days off to rest completely.

Moderate- in this level, the patient has reduced mobility. The daily activities were also restricted and his level of ability varies. This requires longer periods of rest and more likely, you already quit work. The patient also lacks sleep and is usually disturbed.

Severe- the patient can only carry out very minimal tasks like washing her face or brushing her teeth. Likewise, she is having difficulties in concentrating and mental processing. Usually, the patient is also wheelchair-dependent and will only leave home on rare occasions. Likewise, the patient experiences severe after-effects after any activities. Most of their time are spent in bed, sensitive with bright lights and cannot tolerate noise.

These symptoms normally start abruptly. In other cases, patients develop it gradually for weeks or months. Moreover, the symptoms can vary from day to day and tend to stop only to start again. The symptoms of chronic fatigue syndrome covers a broad range but remember the core set of symptoms discussed earlier. These affect almost everyone with the syndrome. Furthermore, others experience a combination of very fast heartbeat, dizziness, light-headedness, urinating often, irritable bowel syndrome, nausea and shortness of breath after an activity.

There are also instances when they feel sweating, low body temperature, appetite and weight change and cold hands and feet. Acquiring depression along with the chronic fatigue syndrome is also very common which only worsen the condition. Only a thorough evaluation one can diagnose the syndrome since its symptoms are very similar to that of other diseases.

The Prognosis

The experience of having chronic fatigue syndrome generally differs from one person to another. However in most cases, the symptoms are bothering and disabling. More often, the patient can experience fluctuation of symptoms during the course of the illness. There will be times that the symptoms are mild and times that it will flare up.

If we are to look at the long-term condition, most patients with chronic fatigue syndrome exhibit improvement especially with therapies and treatment.

While others recover in less than a year, some would stay ill for more years. Nonetheless, the functioning and health of a patient who recovered from CFS do not completely return to its previous levels. In some cases, there are still relapses of the symptoms and may persist for years and those who have been ill for several years are less likely to recover.

Chapter 2: What Is Chronic Fatigue Syndrome?

Millions of people all over the world suffer from chronic fatigue syndrome. Chronic fatigue syndrome is a debilitating disease that is characterized by overwhelming fatigue that is not made better by rest. It is made worse by exercise and mental activity.

Most people who suffer from this syndrome find they are no longer able to function at the activity level they were able to prior to developing this illness. The specific causes are unknown and there are no test to diagnosis it. Since many of the symptoms of seem to overlap, a series of tests must be run to rule out other possible causes.

Chronic Fatigue Syndrome (CFS) is a complex disorder about which little is known. The reasons for onset, etiology or cause of CFS are still largely unknown. In spite of the fact that more than one million individuals suffer from the disorder in the United States alone, physicians are still focused primarily on symptoms, rather than causality.

There are no physical signs to alert an individual or your medical practitioner to the presence of CFS, nor are there any conclusive diagnostic laboratory tests designed to diagnose it. The only thing more difficult than diagnosing and treating chronic fatigue syndrome, is living with it.

The onset

Chronic Fatigue Syndrome differs from other chronic illnesses in that about three-fourths of occurrences come with what can only be described as an abrupt onset, often presenting suddenly and, seemingly, out of nowhere.

Other instances of chronic fatigue spring up after a long period of mild symptoms, generally triggered by a traumatic event or stress. While suggestive, the link between stress and chronic fatigue remains only that...suggestive.

The research into CFS has been extensive, published virtually around the world and in every scientific journal and magazine you can think of, the interest is intense as the disorder reaches epidemic levels. Every organization, from the National Science Foundation (NSF), to the National Institutes of Health (NIH), and the Center for Disease Control (CDC) have researched this complex and puzzling phenomenon, but to no avail.

There are a number of powerful hypotheses but as of yet no solid data to support any of them. While anecdotal, it seems that the disorder only recently, in fact over the past three and one-half decades, has burst onto the scene, peaking the interest of scientists, researchers, and the medical community as a whole.

No solid conclusions have been drawn pertaining to transmission of chronic fatigue. In fact there is no evidence at all to support the proposition that CFS may be contagious. Nevertheless, multiple cases of the disorder have been diagnosed in the same family.

There does seem to be powerful suggestive evidence that chronic fatigue may indeed have a genetic component, however, the jury is still out. More research is needed to prove or disprove the suggestion that CFS is or is not genetic.

Chronic Fatigue Syndrome is categorized by incapacitating, debilitating, and even totally disabling fatigue. CFS presents with a myriad of symptoms, many resembling other illnesses. Symptoms of CFS mimic those of several other disorders, making it extremely difficult to properly diagnose.

Chronic fatigue symptoms are similar to those of Fibromyalgia Syndrome, Myofascial Pain Syndrome, multiple sclerosis, mononucleosis, and even Lyme disease. The symptoms are widespread, and are usually broken down into three categories, they are listed below.

Many sufferers of CFS find it nearly impossible to perform any sort of physical exertion. When engaged in physical activity, such as exercise or any sort of physical labor, the CFS sufferer may experience shortness of breath, light-headedness, and even blackouts.

While some individuals are able to conquer the work week, usually exerting tremendous effort to do so, many more are bedridden, forced to rely solely on others, totally disabled. Problems compound in the ear, nose and throat area, appearing to be endocrine driven symptoms (glands and hormones).

Sore throats and swollen lymph nodes occur, perhaps suggestive of an infection (antigen/antibody reaction), as when the body attempts to fight off a foreign body or when the body is undergoing an extreme stress reaction.

While allergies develop and symptoms become more severe, fevers often present as a symptom as well. Additionally, CFS sufferers will experience night sweats, weight change with little or no apparent change in dietary habits, and they will often suffer from irritable bowel syndrome and bladder dysfunction. Interestingly, many of the conditions listed above are often present during periods of exaggerated stress.

Sleep disorders are a common symptom of CFS and it has been suggested that increased pain sensitivity may contribute to the restlessness and sleeplessness many experience.

Chronic fatigue sufferers often experience difficulty with their senses, mainly in the form of vision changes and sensitivity to bright light, olfactory changes (odor perception) and sensitivity to certain chemicals have been documented.

Disorientation may also occur with CFS, while some suffer with problems of balance and spatial perception. Trouble with concentration and memory have also been reported, seeming to present along with impaired word usage during a phenomenon called "brain fog." Some living with CFS are even subject to seizure-like episodes and unusual and disturbing nightmares.

Depression is often connected with chronic fatigue syndrome. Along with depression, CFS sufferers experience suicidal ideation, anxiety (with or without panic attacks), anger and rage issues, and mood swings ranging from pronounced manic episodes to suicidal depression.

The depression experienced alongside CFS may be chemically induced, due to a serotonin and norepinephrine imbalance, as well as a consequence of external events, such as severe pain, disability, and hopelessness due to lack of treatment options.

CFS varies in degree and expression, type and severity, from one patient to the next. In the same individual, chronic fatigue may wax and wane from one day to the next, even hour to hour. Chronic Fatigue Syndrome symptoms may be mild to acute, fleeting to chronic, in the same individual and from day-to-day.

Chronic Fatigue Syndrome crosses all barriers and touches individuals from all walks of life. There are no clear ethnic, socioeconomic or age-related factors...anyone may be affected. However, there does seem to be a gender issue, with twice as many women as men presenting with the disorder, particularly women between 30 and 50 years of age.

Of the known cases of CFS, those with verifiable diagnoses, at least twice as many women have the disease as men. It also appears to affect pregnant women at a much higher rate than the rest of the population. The reason or reasons for the gender discrepancy, like the difficulty with the initial diagnosis, is problematic and requires more research.

The complexity of the disorder, combined with a lack of any sort of diagnostic standard, results in a medical community that is reactive, required to treat symptoms, with little or no real idea of etiology (cause).

The impact of chronic fatigue on the lives of those suffering from this debilitating and disabling disorder is unfathomable to those who aren't living it on a daily basis.

Like Chronic Pain Syndrome, Chronic Fatigue Syndrome creates a constellation of secondary and tertiary consequences, some as bad if not worse than the original condition. Until etiology (cause) is established, CFS sufferers deal with, on a daily basis, one of the most debilitating of all disorders.

While their load may be lightened with an individually designed and implemented treatment strategy, the ultimate treatment, a cure, still appears elusive.

Women are four times more likely to develop it than men. It usually strikes people between the ages of 40 and 50 but has been diagnosed in some children and teenagers. It is believed that less than 20 percent of CFS suffers have been diagnosed correctly. There continues to be much research done to determine the cause of chronic fatigue syndrome.

There is no known cure for the syndrome. It is believed that the longer diagnosis is delayed the poorer the outcome. Treatment is aimed at relieving the symptoms thru drugs and therapies.

Patients must make many lifestyle changes in order to find what level of activity they can tolerate. Reducing stress, dietary changes and mild stretching appear to help some patients. Medication to promote sleep is often prescribed.

Recovery from chronic fatigue syndrome differs with each patient. Some patients remain home bound. Others recover to the point that they are able to return to work and lead a normal life again, although they continue to have some symptoms.

It is unclear how many patients actually recover but estimates are about 40 percent. Full recovery is rare and estimates are that only about 5-10 percent of patients are symptom free.

Being a mystery to medical science, the chronic fatigue syndrome may have many years but the term was coined only a few decades earlier. Although a growing number of people diagnosed with chronic fatigue syndrome, many people inside and outside the health professions still doubt its existence, or that it is a psychological illness.

Depending on symptoms, chronic fatigue syndrome can make a normal life very difficult. The chronic fatigue syndrome has many symptoms, but most associated with the disease is severe fatigue that makes even get out of bed or difficult to perform normal daily activity.

Persons employed full time have been known to spend months, sometimes years of work, for obvious reasons, it creates a lot of psychological and emotional distress.

Other common symptoms are often found in CFS are suffering: every weakness, sleep disorders, muscle and joint pain, loss of appetite, headache, lymph nodes in the neck or armpit, sore throat, mild fever intestinal problems, anxiety, depression and mental confusion.

Although the cause remains unknown, there is a common factor is that the symptoms of chronic fatigue often occur after a viral infection that is sometimes associated with Epstein-Barr virus.

Many theories are being tested to find the exact cause and some believe is caused by a reaction to specific environmental conditions and chemicals, while others consider the possibility of a collapse of the immune system.

The severity of symptoms that affect each person vary, and so is the effect of the status of CFS patients with certain leaders, while others almost normal existence may be immobilized in bed for several days or the worst case for weeks or months at a time.

As difficult or too heavy are their symptoms, it is important to remember that there are steps you can take to improve your symptoms.

The important factor for people suffering from chronic fatigue syndrome to focus on is to remember that there is a good treatment for fatigue and suffering of many natural therapies and supplements that you can take to increase energy reduce pain, reduce anxiety and depression.

Chapter 3: Metabolism Simplified

Before I can help you educate yourself about what to eat to lose weight and boost energy, you need to grasp one important concept: metabolism. Yes, that word again. You've seen it thousands of times in every health magazine and fad diet book, but do you actually understand what it is? It's important to learn about your metabolism because it's directly affected by what you eat.

To sum up metabolism in one basic statement, it is a group of processes that manage your fuel. Imagine that your body is a car. Much like a car, your body runs on fuel. You fill up your car with gas, just as you feed your body with food. Think of the act of driving as the car's metabolism. Only metabolism, as it is related to your body, is not quite as simple. Your metabolism gets your body going, so to speak, and since the human body does many things simultaneously, the processes that make up your metabolism are complex and continuous.

Did you know that even as you sit and read, your metabolism is hard at work and therefore, you're burning calories? You're probably thinking, "If that's true, then why am I not losing more weight?" Well, the rate at which your metabolism burns calories depends on many factors. Your genes may impact your metabolic rate; some people just burn through fuel much faster than others. They also usually have more energy as a result, because a faster metabolism means an increase in energy. That being said, despite your genetic makeup, other factors that determine your metabolic rate are very much in your control.

One such factor is your food intake. What you eat affects your metabolic rate, which in turn affects how much of your food is stored as energy in your fat cells and how quickly it is used to fuel your body's functions and activities. Your metabolic rate can be broken down into three parts: the Basal Metabolic Rate (BMR), energy burned through physical activity, and the thermic effect of food. Your Basal Metabolic Rate is the rate at which your metabolism burns energy just to fuel your body's functions. In other words, this is the energy that's burned while you're not physically active. Your BMR equals 50 to 80 percent of the energy that is used by your metabolism. The energy that is used during physical activity is pretty straight forward, as you may imagine. That's the energy that is burned during movement, but, surprisingly, it only contributes around 20 percent of the energy used by your metabolism. The thermic effect of food is the energy that is burned during your consumption and digestion of food. In other words, you use fuel to refuel and distribute that new intake of fuel.

The bottom line is that most of the energy used by your metabolism goes toward fueling your body's most basic functions.

You don't burn most of your energy through physical movement, though you can increase the energy you burn through physical activity, depending on the vigorousness of the activity you perform. Also, you actually need to use energy to gain more energy. The point being that exercise isn't the simple answer for speeding up your metabolism, contrary to popular belief. Food, however, has a very profound impact because it determines how much energy will be used to digest it, and how much energy will be stored in your fat cells. The idea is to increase your BMR, and though you can't control your BMR directly like you can control your energy use during physical activity, the food you digest can help boost your BMR, hence, boosting your energy.

Let's uncover some truths about the human metabolism. Do you ever wonder why your husband can eat a scrumptious-looking dessert in addition to a hearty meal and not gain a pound, while you seem to visibly expand after eating the same thing? The simple yet unfortunate fact is that men tend to have faster metabolisms than women. Generally, males have larger, more muscular bodies than females, and larger bodies use more energy with their BMR. Also, the more muscle you have, the larger your BMR is and the faster your overall metabolism becomes. Another rather unwelcome fact is metabolism slows down with age. Chances are you've heard this before countless times, but the reason for it is still a mystery to you. It's simple; the more muscle you have, the faster your metabolism is, because you're BMR mostly uses your muscles to burn energy. As you get older, your body loses muscle, causing a decrease in energy usage through your BMR. It isn't necessarily true that thinner people have a faster metabolism. As noted before, a larger person has a more active BMR, and that can extend to people who are overweight and obese. The partiality to that truth is that more calories are burned when a person is muscular, and when you have a lot of body fat it most likely exceeds your amount of muscle, so your metabolism is still limited.

Do you ever feel horribly tired even if you haven't exerted yourself much throughout the day? Of course, the busy schedule that comes with being a wife, mother and a career woman runs you ragged on a regular basis, but there are probably some days that have been comparatively slower, and yet you still feel fatigued. I felt that way on weekends. We would drive up to our lake house for a couple of days, and even though the kids stayed outside most of the time and ate boxed lunches, I felt like a worn-out rag by bedtime. The hubby would always complain that I was too tired to even watch a movie on TV during those trips. Well, I learned that a lower BMR can definitely cause that sort of fatigue.

Those countless fad diets you've embarked on over the years may have wreaked some havoc with your overall metabolism, though recent research shows that so-called yo-yo dieting does not permanently slow it down. Still, here's why those diets never worked, and why your weight kept fluctuating with each attempt. Surprise, surprise: It has everything to do with your metabolism. Many of those diets have no doubt promoted restricting your caloric intake to an extreme degree. Sure, it makes sense that the less active you are, the less calories you need to function, but again, it's not so clear-cut. Since your BMR is the component of your metabolism that burns the energy used to maintain your body, you need a higher BMR to gain energy and lose weight. Yet if your caloric intake decreases, so does your BMR, so you can't achieve the goal of losing weight. You lose the most weight in the beginning of a diet pattern because, as a person with fat to burn, your metabolism is higher than it would be if you were not overweight. But as your caloric intake decreases, your metabolism slows, and the pounds are free to cling to you like leeches. Therefore, the idea is not to eat fewer calories, but to get your calories from a variety of choices. No, this doesn't mean that you should sit down to dinner and eat a meal consisting of a double chicken sandwich, a pile of steak fries and a milkshake, a meal worth thousands of calories. (Not that I'd ever do that myself, of course!) Over time, I learned that you are better off eating a moderate meal made up of food that is healthier, more natural and, therefore, more friendly toward your digestive system and metabolism.

Chapter 4: Diet – What To Eat To Look And Feel Good

The first thing you need to do to battle fatigue is to evaluate and change your diet. There is a lot of misconception about the word "diet." A diet isn't some weight-loss program; it's actually much simpler and broader than that. A diet is simply everything you consume during the day, such as meals, snacks and beverages. If you eat pizza for breakfast, Chinese takeout for lunch and burgers for dinner, that's your diet. Diets can be healthy or unhealthy, and, in order to battle fatigue, you'll need the right foods in your diet to give your body the proper nutrients to function.

Leafy Green Vegetables

Leafy green vegetables are high in essential vitamins and minerals, such as iron, vitamin E and folate. Leafy green vegetables also contain fiber, which helps keep you full during the day and prevents you from snacking on junk food that only depletes your energy. A few common leafy green vegetables you can include in your diet are:

- Collard greens
- Spinach
- Kale
- Swiss chard
- Romaine lettuce
- Arugula

Nuts

Raw nuts are perfect snack food to help boost your energy throughout the day. The energy-giving ingredient in nuts is protein, and this healthy nutrient is what will help you feel more energized during the day. Some nuts also contain magnesium, which is a key mineral that turns sugar in your body into energy. Pack a small snack bag or box of any type nuts, and take it with you everywhere you go to have a little pick-me-up snack. Here are a few healthy types of nuts that you can munch on:

☐ Almonds

☐ Cashews

☐ Walnuts

☐ Hazelnuts

☐ Pecans

Hydration

Fueling your body with water is another way to energize yourself and battle fatigue. Even though it's recommended that you drink eight regular glasses of water each day, you can also get water from food and use food to get a healthy water consumption. These foods include:

☐ Fruits – melons, strawberries, apples, oranges

☐ Cucumbers

- [ ] Bell peppers
- [ ] Lettuce

Chapter 5: Understanding The Stressors In The Modern Workplace

Today's modern workers are on the constant lookout for ways to achieve work-life balance. The very concept itself negates a close examination of the time you usually spend at work as opposed to the time you allot for personal development and recreation. Ideally, one should not supersede the other. This means that you should be able to achieve a sense of professional stability without affecting the quality of your life, and vice versa. Failure to achieve this balance denotes a disproportionate allocation of time and resources for one thing at the expense of the other.

The ultimate question therefore is: Is this so-called work-life balance ever achievable? If so, how can you achieve it? If not, what could be tapped in place of it?

First off, it is important to recognize the state of the modern workplace. A lot has definitely changed since the olden days, more so with the advent of technological innovations, the shifting dynamics of the global marketplace, and the highs and lows of the economic landscape. Needless to say, the way things are done these days are far different from the traditional methods. As such, the modern workplace requires workers who are adept at multiple skills, ready to spend long hours at work, available for contact 24/7, and highly proficient to a set of unique tasks and responsibilities.

Uncertain economy

Compounding the plight of today's workers are the continuing challenges posed by a weak, almost uncertain, economy. Job security is an issue that many people are secretly wary of, given the spate of mass layoffs and budget cuts that remain prevalent to this day. Consequently, the national unemployment rate hovers at a dangerous figure, with more people looking for jobs that aren't simply there. Those who managed to keep their jobs, on the other hand, opt to clock in more work hours in the hopes of shielding themselves from the risks of being laid off.

Beyond the workplace lies the equally vibrant and demanding social arena where workers spend the other half of their day. In this setting, workers have to deal with their families, friends, loved ones, kids, as well as their personal aspirations and goals. When this setting is juxtaposed against the demands of the modern workplace, you get a chaotic loop of tasks, demands, and challenges that can only be untangled if you have a firm grasp of proper stress and time management.

Physical, mental, and emotional exhaustion

Admittedly, the constancy of pressure, stress, and the rigid demands of both your professional and personal life can be a little challenging to deal with all at the same time. This is precisely the reason why those who are unable to sufficiently cope with these things find themselves getting burned out. Not only does getting burned out affect you negatively on an emotional and mental level, it also manifests itself by posing adverse effects to your physical state. Worse, when left unchecked, it can also branch out to your relationships with other people, including your family, friends, and colleagues at work.

Thankfully, achieving work-life balance is not an entirely impossible task. There are in fact strategies and techniques that you can employ in your day to day activities to help you overcome the challenges posed by the demands and stresses of your life.

In the end, keep in mind that you don't have to sacrifice one aspect of your life in favor of the other. All it takes is to find the sustainable balance between your career and your personal life. The succeeding chapters provide a detailed exploration of the various methods that you can use to kick start your quest for a better quality of life.

Chapter 6: Get A Schedule

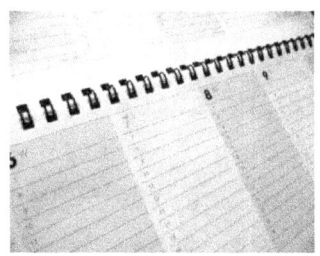

The National Sleep Foundation recommends that you stick to a regular bedtime routine. That means going to sleep and waking up at the same time every day (yes, even weekends!). Try to avoid spending more time in bed than you need. Maintaining good light hygiene will help: Open the blinds or go outside as soon as you wake to get energized, and shut off all the lights (including electronics) when you go to sleep. Wake up at the same time each day. It is tempting to sleep late on weekends, especially if you have had poor sleep during the week. However, if you suffer from insomnia or sleeping problems, you should get up at the same time every day in order to train your body to wake at a consistent time. I know for some this can be hard. We all have unpredictable schedules at times, or you may do shift work for your job, or even have a very active social life, but whatever the situation, it is important to do your best to get into a good schedule to train our circadian biological clock. Most people notice that they naturally experience different levels of sleepiness and alertness throughout the day, but what causes these patterns? Sleep is regulated by two body systems: sleep/wake homeostasis and the circadian biological clock. When we have been awake for a long period of time, sleep/wake homeostasis tells us that a need for sleep is accumulating and that it is time to sleep. It also helps us maintain enough sleep throughout the night to make up for the hours of being awake. If this restorative process existed alone, it would mean that we would be most alert as our day was starting out, and that the longer we were awake, the more we would feel like sleeping. In this way, sleep/wake homeostasis creates a drive that balances sleep and wakefulness. Our internal circadian biological clocks, on the other hand, regulates the timing of periods of sleepiness and wakefulness throughout the day. The circadian rhythm dips and rises at different times of the day, so adults' strongest sleep drive generally occurs between 2:00-4:00 am and in the afternoon between 1:00-3:00 pm, although there is some variation depending on whether you are a "morning person" or "evening person." So by getting into a good schedule, you can help your body produce the melatonin at the right times, allowing you to fall asleep at the right time and wake up feeling refreshed, which will allowing you to be productive throughout the day. Now let's move on to what you can do throughout the day because it will influence what happens at night. It may seem silly to prepare throughout the day for sleeping at night time, but preparation is what makes the winners. Or as Benjamin Franklin put it, "By failing to prepare, you are preparing to fail".

Chapter 7: Back To Basics

TAPPING

It appears that most people in the western world are always on the run. Busy running around to take care of their family, or busy at work, or getting stuck in traffic going to and from work, business meetings, and so on. We are so busy taking care of everything else and everyone else that we don't seem to have the time to take better care of ourselves.

I'd like to share some simple techniques that do not take much time which you can start using today on yourself.

Tapping is a fun method that works best the moment you wake up.

Put your feet on the floor while sitting on your bed and start to tap the top of your head and yawning. Then tap the sides of your head and the back of your neck and finally the front of your head and gently around your face and eyes.

Next start tapping one arm and then the opposite arm and the entire front of the chest. Continue to tap the front of your legs and top of each foot and the bottom of both feet.

What this does is increase the blood flow and oxygen throughout your body which makes you much more alert and ready to start your day.

TOTAL TIME IS ABOUT 3 - MINUTES

When oxygen levels are increased, the red blood cells pick up the extra oxygen, and provide it to our body tissues. Waste gases and toxins are removed more efficiently and cells begin to function normally. Anaerobic viruses, bacteria and fungi, unable to live in an oxygen enriched environment, are compromised. Oxygen builds resistance to infections like yeast (candida albicans) that thrive in an oxygen deficient environment. Oxygen helps to neutralize acids in our body, like lactic acid resulting from muscle overload. Our body's chemical reactions are 'fired-up' due to the increased oxygen levels. We burn fat more efficiently. We feel better, our body is healthier and we think more clearly because of increased oxygenation.

Tapping is just one way you can keep your body moving. Other alternatives are:

Chewing gum

Flexing your hands

Moving your neck from side to side

Flexing and contracting your feet

Rotating your wrists

Standing up and taking a walk during your coffee break

B.E.S.T

RELEASE STRESS/CLEARING EMOTIONAL DRAMA WITH EASE

This first system call B.E.S.T – Bio-Energetic Synchronization Technique is something that must be done by a B.E.S.T Practitioner but it's worth its weight in gold. This system is based on active healing and removing interference from the body so the body can heal itself.

While lying on a table face up or face down, the Practitioner uses gentle touch on various parts of the body to receive messages. It's so profound that I was cleared from a blockage in my left leg related to a car accident I'd been in 30 years prior.

Once a month or so, I would have stiffness and pain in that same area but using this method cleared it. I haven't had any pain or stiffness since this treatment and that was six months ago.

In my next B.E.S.T. treatment, we cleared fear based memories from my childhood that I'd completely forgotten about but showed up to be faced in the light of day.

Interesting enough, it cleared guilt and worthiness issues. Within a month of that clearing, I returned to my Kentucky home for a face to face visit with a man that had abused me as a child. I looked at him and felt nothing but

The first week of January I ask Lynne to do a couple of treatments with my vision board. (A Vision board consist of a group of pictures showing things you want to do in the future. Like traveling, or new adventures, or a new home etc.)

Here it is now in June, six months later and all the things on my vision board have happened with such ease I almost forgot about it.

My vision board had pictures of beautiful kitchens and baths along with a new car. My kitchen and bath have been updated with granite and cabinets similar to the pictures I posted. And my new car is even more beautiful than the one in the photo. If that's not enough the money showed up as a tax refund that covered all of my expenses. I love these synchronicities.

I have since then sent several people to experience Lynne's amazing work and their lives have changed in wonderful ways. Lynne Webb is an ELITE MASTER B.E.S.T PRACTITIONER. To find one near your area visit www.morter.com

To Contact Lynne Webb: call (1-949-533-2384)

In Lynne's office, she has these products that hold Ancient Codes and can truly transform your life. They are called "I-Ching Systems".

I-CHING SYSTEMS

These personal transforming products, some of which you place your hands on, others you place in a room, others you put your feet on, and there are other ones made specifically for you. I had the opportunity to go to a seminar where I experienced all these products with a group of friends and by the end of the weekend, we all felt a shift in our body temple. Two months after this experience, we all had amazing doors of change opened to us. It's indeed a beautiful thing for you to experience.

Below are sample products from I-Ching systems.

PERFECT BALANCE CARD is used for emotional balance. Some people carry it in their purses at work and have noticed amazing transformation in their work place just having it with them. You can also place your hands on it for 10-15 minutes when you've had a stressful situation as it calms you down, gives clarity and gets you going. This card contains ancient symbols and rely on many principles found in acupuncture.

QUIET PLEASE CARD is designed to quiet your mind especially at the end of the day when you are preparing to sleep. Anyone of any age bracket can use this card. You can put it around your neck as it helps you stay calm and focused. I am wearing one as I write this book so I don't get distracted from the task in front of me. It's amazing.

BALANCE SPACE SYMBOL CARD can be hung on a wall of your home or business. It's based on the principles of Feng Shui, the ancient system for balancing the energies in an environment. It's been used in Therapist office and clients have lost the urge to drink alcohol.

My friends and clients notice how calm they feel when they visit my home or my office within minutes. It's great to have in a home that's chaotic or has a lot of emotional drama going on. I wish this had been around when I was growing up.

These are just a few of the products from I-Chings Systems. For more information

Visit - www.ichingsystemsinstruments.com or call Mary Miller at (1-508-944-4250)

Tell her Ella the Author sent you.

Chapter 8: What Is Occupational Burnout?

Do you know that feeling when you do something so much that you get sick of it? Well, that's the shortest explanation of occupational burnout.

Work burnout, as it's also known, is a condition characterized by exhaustion. It might be physical, emotional, intellectual, or all of them together. One feels drained and empty, with no energy or will for work. It occurs due to prolonged work-related stress and affects one's life in many ways.

Burnout is not an official medical diagnosis, but according to some experts, there are other conditions behind burnout, such as depression. Many people who experience burnout don't even believe that their job is the main cause.

Official diagnosis or not, occupational burnout can majorly affect your physical and mental health. That's why it is important to recognize if you're experiencing occupational burnout and then consider how to recover from it.

How to Tell If You're Suffering from Burnout

Do any of the following sound familiar?

You feel a constant lack of energy.

Your sleeping habits have changed. You sleep the whole day, or have trouble falling or staying asleep.

You have to force yourself to go to work and it's tough for you to get started.

You've become impatient and irritable with people around you, especially at work—co-workers, clients, and customers.

You've become critical and cynical about work and people at work.

You lack the energy to be as productive as you need to.

It's hard for you to concentrate and stay focused.

You don't care about your achievements anymore; they no longer bring you joy.

You have no more illusions or passion for your job.

You're are using food to feel better.

You're using alcohol or drugs to feel better or to not think about what's bothering you.

You suffer from headaches.

You experience unexplained stomach or intestinal problems, or other random pain.

If any of the above refers to you, you might be experiencing job burnout. First, you need to see a doctor or a mental health provider to rule out other possible causes. If there's no other diagnosis or condition provoking it, chances are your job is the element out of balance.

Although it's not an official medical diagnosis, that doesn't mean it's not dangerous. Occupational burnout is not something you should have to live with. That sense of emptiness and exhaustion is not normal. There are many things that can help you recover and bring back your energy and life satisfaction.

Possible Causes and Risk Factors

Before we start searching for the solutions to our problems, most of us like to know what causes them in the first place. And it makes sense: if you know the source of your troubles, you can eliminate it or at least minimize its impact.

So what could be the cause of occupational burnout?

Job burnout is not the same as stress from work. Stress is a normal part of our daily lives and careers, and it won't cause damage if it's managed well. But if you are constantly exposed to high levels of stress and do nothing about mitigating it, it will lead to burnout.

If your job consumes so much of your energy that you don't have time for family, friends, and other things that make your personal life fulfilling, you'll burn out quickly.

Social isolation at work and in your personal life is a risk factor for many kinds of mental health issues. Job burnout is not an exception. If you feel isolated, you'll experience higher levels of stress and be more prone to burnout.

When a job is chaotic or monotonous, you need more energy to stay focused. This drains you, creating higher levels of stress leading to adrenal fatigue and occupational burnout.

If you feel undermined by colleagues, unappreciated by your boss, or you work with an office bully or other kind of toxic co-worker, it won't be enough to love your job. We all need to feel accepted and connected, and our workplace is not an exception. If you work with people and don't feel good in their company, it drains your energy and sets you on the path to burnout.

If you are not clear about what your duty is, what level of authority you have, and what others expect from you, you can't feel comfortable. It can be particularly stressful trying to meet someone else's expectations when you don't even know what they are. If you lack feedback, you can't know if you are on the right path, which makes the stress worse.

If you have no influence on decisions that affect your job, such as workload, schedule, and assignments, or you don't have enough resources to complete the job, you might feel powerless and stressed. This feeling of not being in control of things that affect your life leads to burnout, too.

Almost anyone can experience occupational burnout at some point in life. However, there are some factors that could make you more likely to experience it. Here are some of them:

Your job is to help people. Employees in the service professions, such as the health care sector, are more prone to burnout.

You work A LOT. High workload, a busy schedule, and overtime hours are risk factors for job burnout.

You identify with your work. If you do this and neglect your personal life, it creates an imbalance, which leads to burnout.

You are doing too much on your own. If you try to do everything by yourself, it's time to learn how to delegate. Also, if you don't set healthy boundaries and try to be there for everyone, you are at high risk.

You have too little impact and control over your work. Someone else is in charge of your schedule, workload, and assignments.

You find your job to be dull and monotonous.

You feel lonely and isolated at your workplace or in your personal in life.

What If You Do Nothing About It?

Occupational burnout is not an illness, it's a condition. It's not a medical diagnosis, but that doesn't mean it can't lead to some serious health and mental issues. You might think it's not your job that causes you to feel like this. Or you think you are just tired, you need a rest, some time away from work, and everything will fall back into place.

There is some truth in this. It's not only your job that causes the problem; you really need rest and some time away from your duties. But this is not all. A vacation, even a terrific one, won't fix things completely. Job burnout didn't happen overnight. So it's not realistic to expect it to disappear just like that. Recovery will take time and effort.

If you don't address or try to ignore job burnout, the only thing you can expect is for it to get worse and cause additional problems.

This might include:

More and more stress

Chronic fatigue

Sleeping problems, insomnia

Sadness and depression

Anxiety and panic

Irritability, outbursts of anger, and problems controlling your rage

Alcohol abuse

Drug use

High blood pressure

Heart disease

Type 2 diabetes

Low immune system and vulnerability to illnesses

Problems in personal interactions

Lower quality of life in general

These are just some of the consequences if occupational burnout goes unaddressed and is not confronted. Obviously, it's a serious condition that requires you to take it seriously and do whatever is in your power to solve it. Last but not least, you have only one life. Do you really want to spend it tired, grumpy, cynical, and desperate?

Chapter 9: Intestinal Support

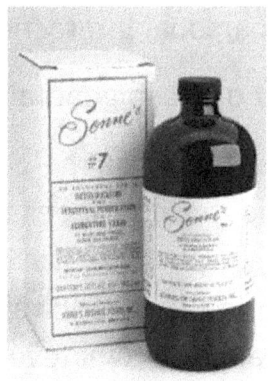

On a colon cleanse day, eat very little. Liquids would be best for 24 hours.

I started with a very gentle colon cleanse using Bernard Jensen's technique. Today, everyone and her/his mother is selling colon cleanse kits which are very expensive and contain too many ingredients for the chemically sensitive individual. Use Sonne's #7 (Bentonite solution) and Sonne's #9 (Psyllium powder.)

In a bottle with a screw top:

· Mix 1 tablespoon Bentonite (Sonne's #7) liquid with 1 tablespoon (Sonne's #9) Psyllium powder, in 8 oz. of clean filtered water. If you cannot find Sonne's products, you may substitute another brand of Bentonite and Psyllium.
· Shake it vigorously for 15 seconds.
· Drink it all.

Since I was not able to eat many foods, I shed black sausage-like casings in the shape of intestines. I took photos of it because I couldn't believe it! This is called the mucoid layer or plaque.

LEAKY GUT

How do I know if I have it? You can take expensive tests or realize that if you are chronically ill, you probably have it!

What do I do? First, you must clean up your diet. No gluten for the time being; no dairy except butter or ghee; no sugar; no yeast products, no allergenic foods, and you must be on a rotation diet. Read every label.

L-Glutamine is the nutrient known for healing a leaky gut. There will be some people who will become too excited on the supplement. If so, discontinue.

Order a pure glutamine powder that dissolves in water and drink first thing in the morning. Continue for 2-3 months and then get off of it.

There are many books written just on gut immunity. I like to address gut immunity using l-glutamine, colostrum, Immunoglobulins, lactoferrin, probiotics and digestive enzymes.

an important thing to remember when detoxing...

The liver will dump toxins to the small intestines, then to the large intestine to be excreted through the sigmoid colon followed by a bowel movement. In order to not reabsorb these toxins back into your body, one needs to BIND them. I cannot tell you how important it is to use a binder.

Some people use psyllium, bentonite, zeolite, or other clays, but the product I have found on the market that is best tolerated and effective is called "BIND" by Systemic Formulas. I would not be without it. Take 3 capsules, twice a day between meals. For people who have mycotoxins and by-products of microbes (yes, microbes crap in us!), this is an essential step.

No drainage, no detox!

I used liver drainages as well. There is a saying, "Detox without drainage is suicide." I tested for whatever homeopathic extracts my body wanted. Test your body. There so many liver drainages on the market.

h. (HELIOBACTOR) pYLORI

A genetic test is the only test that can accurately diagnose H. Pylori. The breath test and the blood test produce too many false negatives.

My physician touched the upper part of my intestine right under the ribs and I screamed. He said," I think you have H. Pylori". I took a breath test that was negative. I took a blood test where only IgA was positive. The results were inconclusive. So I did an experiment with Gum Mastica and Gastromycin to see if any symptoms of H.Pylori would occur.

Gum Mastica starts the process of killing and releasing H.Pylori while Bismuth in the supplement, Gastromycin, cleans it up from the stomach lining. H. Pylori likes to hang on. If you have a serious ulcer from H. Pylori, please visit a Functional Medicine doctor.

Start with two Gum Mastica in the morning on an empty stomach and two at night, on an empty stomach for 2-3 months. At first you may get a pain in the pit of your stomach after taking two Gum Mastica, but Gastromycin will stop the pain while killing the H. Pylori that are clinging to the stomach wall.

Take Gastromycin 4 caps with meals, twice a day.

Bismuth, is a necessary but a toxic substance that you will use only for two weeks. Pepto-Bismol has bismuth in it. Some people take Pepto-Bismol because they don't tolerate Gastromycin. If the pain in the upper part of your stomach goes away, then the bismuth is killing the H. Pylori that is notorious for clinging to the stomach wall. I did not take any antibiotics at all.

There are individuals who eat fermented foods, whether bought or home-made, to address SIBO (Small Intestinal Bacteria Overload). I never felt that fermented vegetables helped me, although I eat raw sauerkraut.

Chapter 10: How Much Energy We Need Daily

What are the approximated calories we need daily

The following calorie requirement chart presents probable amounts of calorie consumption required to maintain the power balance to get more power and a healthy body weight for various sex and age groups at three different stages of exercising. The estimates are rounded to the nearest 200 calorie consumption and were identified using an equation from the Institute of Medicine (IOM).

Estimated calorie specifications (in kilocalories) for each gender and age team at three stages of actual action.

• These stages are depending on Estimated Energy Specifications (EER) from the IOM Dietary Referrals Intakes macronutrients report, 2002, calculated by sex, age, and activity stage for reference-sized individuals. "Reference size," as identified by IOM, is depending on the average size for age groups up to age 18 years old and average size of that size to give a BMI of 21.5 for women and 22.5 for males.

• Sedentary indicates a way of lifestyle that contains only the mild exercising associated with common day-to-day lifestyle.

• Moderately effective indicates a way of lifestyle that contains exercising comparative to strolling about 1.5-3 kilometers per day at 3-4 mph, moreover to the slight exercising associated with day-to-day lifestyle.

• Active indicates a way of lifestyle that contains exercising comparative to strolling more than 3 kilometers per day at 3-4 mph, moreover to the slight exercising associated with day-to-day lifestyle.

- The calorie ranges exposed are to accommodate needs of different age groups within the team. For children and adolescents, more calorie consumption is required for mature age groups. For adults, fewer calorie consumption is required for mature age groups.

Chapter 11: Fatigue Fighting Vitamins And Herbs

Fatigue is mental and physical tiredness where the individual has no vitality or eagerness to do anything. Fatigue is frequently the aftereffect of constant disease, push, workaholic behavior, stress or times of passionate change. It can be the side effect of numerous sicknesses, including paleness and contaminations. Endless fatigue can be enormously enhanced by eating nourishments that expansion the vitality level and bolster the resistant framework. Expelling the development of poisons from the body will decrease the vitality deplete and stretch diminishment strategies may facilitate the indications. Tender practice will fortify the muscles and animate the course and the generation of antibodies to build imperviousness to disease.

What to do about fatigue

As enticing as it is to do nothing when you feel extremely drained or depleted, it is critical to make a move. Here is a basic rundown of things you can use to help assuage and turn around your fatigue.

Vitamins

The vitamins and minerals sketched out beneath can be acquired as a piece of a quality, balanced vitamin and mineral supplement. The balance of these vitamins and minerals is essential as an excess of one can hinder the ingestion or use by the body of another - in this way bringing about an inadequacy.

Vitamin A fortifies the insusceptible framework and battles contaminations. It additionally assumes an imperative part all in all recuperating.

Vitamin B1 enhances the sensory system capacity and lifts vitality. It is basic for changing over nourishment into vitality and for the transmission of electrical driving forces in the nerves and muscles. It can powerfully affect your state of mind and readiness.

Vitamin B6 expands vitality levels. It is basic for the breakdown of nourishment and the creation of vitality in the body. It is additionally vital for the development of antibodies.

Pantothenic corrosive diminishes fatigue and soothes stretch. It is fundamental for the change of sustenance into vitality and for the breakdown of fats.

Folic corrosive is expected to frame sound red platelets which are indispensable for vitality as they convey oxygen to the muscles. It is basic for the digestion system of proteins and sugars.

Vitamin C detoxifies the body and in the process makes vitality more accessible. It helps the body retain press and folic corrosive successfully and transform sustenance into vitality.

Vitamin E bolsters the insusceptible framework. It is an effective cell reinforcement and is imperative for the creation of vitality from sustenance.

Minerals

Calcium is required for the muscles and nerves and enhances rest.

Press diminishes fatigue that is related with inadequate red platelets. It is expected to discharge the vitality in your body. It is likewise basic in keeping up a solid safe framework.

Magnesium decreases shortcoming and tiredness. It is fundamental for transforming nourishment into vitality. The sensory system depends on magnesium to work legitimately and it is esteemed for its anxiety soothing properties.

Selenium is a hostile to oxidant that decreases the vitality deplete created by free radicals. It is basic in keeping an extensive variety of infections. It is required for sound muscles including those of the heart. It helps the invulnerable framework, expanding your capacity to battle contamination.

Zinc aids the detoxification of the body and furthermore helps the safe framework. It is vital for the mind and sensory system and mental sharpness.

Different supplements and herbs

Omega 3 unsaturated fats support vitality.

Acidophilus and other amicable microorganisms help to make a typical intestinal balance. This is essential for enhancing vitality if an excess of Candida is thought to be an issue.

Bioflavonoids upgrade the activity of vitamin C.

Co-compound Q10 expands oxygen take-up in the cells and this can build vitality.

Ginger and Siberian ginseng are herbs that if taken inside will expand your vitality and balance stomach related and hormonal frameworks.

Ginger, red ginseng root, cardamom seed, artichoke leaf and gentian root are herbs for the stomach related framework. Stomach related reinforcing herbs increment your capacity to process sustenance to discharge the vitality from the nourishment that you eat.

Mate and green tea can give a transitory lift in vitality.

Rosemary basic oil (3-4 drops) added to a shower is a decent lift me-up.

Sustenances to eat

The accompanying sustenances will help you get a lift of vitality that is accomplished sustainedly and not only the transient settle that is given by sugar and caffeine which exacerbate you feel later. Do whatever it takes not to gorge.

A lot of new foods grown from the ground, verdant vegetables.

Entire grains, nuts and seeds.

Chicken and fish.

You have to keep away from any wellsprings of sustenance hypersensitivities from your diet, especially wheat and dairy items. You likewise need to stay away from liquor, smoking, refined nourishments and sugars and caffeine. These nourishments exhaust your vitality levels. Keep in mind, cakes, cakes, bread, to be sure anything produced using flour, are altogether refined sustenances. Eating the correct sustenances will lessen the poisons that are put into your body, in any case, it is plausible that your body is now over-burden and you have to purify your colon with the goal that you can rid the body of its lethal load. Poisons are one of the principle explanations behind a lessening in vitality. This is on the grounds that the body's assets must be occupied into managing the undesirable material. To find more about how you can manage poisons, scrub your colon securely and advantage from the expansion in vitality go to safecoloncleansing.com

While you are purifying you likewise need to drink a lot of separated water - so that the body can flush out the poisons.

Home grown cures

There are two home grown cures that can give you a more characteristic profound vitality. You can without much of a stretch make these home grown medications yourself on the off chance that you have the fixings.

For the principal, utilize 1 to 2 teaspoonsful of the accompanying mix.

1 section asparagus root

1 section ginger rhizome

1 section red ginseng root

1 glass water

For the second, add the herbs as indicated by the accompanying.

1 section ginger rhizome

1 section cardamon seeds

1 section artichoke clears out

1/2 section genetian root

1 glass water

For each of them, place the water into a fittingly measured pan and convey to the bubble. Add the herbs to the bubbling water, kill the warmth and permit to remain for 10-15 minutes then strain the blend.

Drink a measure of the blend up to three times each day.

Work out

Regardless of the possibility that you feel tired, attempt to in any event take short strolls in the outside air and work on breathing where it counts into your lungs as you walk. Stroll no less than 20 - 30 minutes for each day, however do begin with shorter periods on the off chance that you have to. The critical thing is to begin getting exercise. Step by step work up to longer and more incessant work out, if conceivable including 20 minutes of oxygen consuming activity each other day.

Stopped Smoking

On the off chance that you smoke you have to stop. Smoking is a noteworthy deplete on your wellbeing and vitality and can undermine every one of your endeavors in different regions. The Growerz.com quit smoking system can help you to end up smoke free.

Attempt to join the same number of these things into your way of life as you are capable. Work out an arrangement for yourself about how you will deal with your day and what you will accomplish in it. While the above points of interest are proposed to be for the most part accommodating and instructive they ought not be interpreted as a substitution for individual counsel from a wellbeing proficient. You ought to look for expert help if your fatigue is sudden, outrageous, durable or you neglect to move forward.

Chapter 12: The Day I Got Sick

My girlfriend and I drove down to Geelong to see the comedians Hale and Pace and to stay for my Mum's birthday. It felt like I had a cold coming on, but I didn't care. The cold symptoms got worse, however, as we sat down in the foyer to watch the comedy show. Still, I didn't think anything more of it than that I would be sick for a short amount of time, but I would be fine in a few days. Halfway through the show, though, I just wasn't laughing as much as I usually would. This cold felt a lot stranger then usual. As soon as the show finished, we drove to my Mum's place to drop off some flowers and a present for her. I had work the next day, so we had to drive back to Melbourne City, which is one hour away from where we were. About ten minutes into driving back home,I I told my girlfriend that I legitimately felt like passing out. I kept saying to her, "I feel really, really sick!" I struggled to drive home, and as soon as we arrived, I just remember collapsing on the bed. It seemed to get worse and worse, and I said to my girlfriend, "Something is very wrong." My throat started to close up to the point where it was half closed. It was like a sore throat times 20. I thought I would be okay, but it kept closing up, and I began to feel even worse. My girlfriend suggested that I go to the hospital but i thought, "No, it cant be that bad." As it got worse, I had no option but to go to the hospital. They gave me numbing gel for my very sore throat and told me there was nothing they could really do. I didn't sleep at all, and I felt so horrible and could barely breathe out of my mouth. For someone who has hay fever, having a blocked nose isn't uncommon, but this was much worse, and I started to panic a little. The following day, I felt even worse than I had the day before, and my throat closed up completely. I could no longer breathe through my mouth, and I could only breathe through one nostril. My girlfriend and I drove out to the doctor because I felt like I was going to die. As I was waiting, I was hyperventilating through my nose as I kept thinking, "If my nose blocks up, I'm going to stop breathing!" I saw the doctor, and he basically just told me to go home. I told him I couldn't breathe and that I needed help, but he didn't believe me, so I left and sat down outside until my friend arrived. I waited for five minutes. I was crying and shaking, and it wasn't until my friend complained and the doctor HAD TO SEE ME that he finally put me on some steroid inhalant. Within 5 minutes, it opened up my throat, and I could breathe again. It was the most horrible experience I have ever experienced in my life. It only lasted about an hour in total but an hour basically fighting to stay alive isn't that much fun. I still had a lot of trouble breathing because of the swelling, but it was enough for me to relax a little more.

He took my blood that day, and I returned about four days later, and he said I had Glandular Fever. All I needed to do was rest, and I would be okay.

The fatigue was unbearable. As weeks went on, I couldn't even leave the bed. It was like there was a 500kg weight holding me down. I will never forget the three months I had to go through this. I used to lie in bed and cry because I couldn't even move my finger. You may be reading this thinking, "Come on, its not that hard to move your fingers!" However, many of you will understand where I am coming from. I would be in bed for four hours, not being able to move any part of my body, and the fatigue was so bad that I found it difficult to breathe. How did I go to the toilet, then? Well, I used to hold it in for ages! I used to find enough strength inside of me to be able to get out of bed only once in a while. Just getting out of the bed and going to the toilet felt like I had just run a 100 mile marathon, and just after the finish line I collapsed. I couldn't even stand up when I went to the toilet; I had to sit down to urinate. I would then just sit there for one or two hours sometimes, because I couldn't move. I would find a little strength again, wash my hands, and often would collapse just before I got back to the bed. There were several times when I would try get out of bed, take about five steps, and then collapse on the floor. My girlfriend was in the lounge room, which was about three meters away from the hallway outside of my bedroom. I was so fatigued that I couldn't even talk to her to let her know I had collapsed. I couldn't even tap on the wall or call for her name. I would lay there and just have tears coming out of my eyes and rolling down my face. 30 minutes would go by, and I would somehow find enough strength to pick myself up and walk the four meters back to bed and, once again, collapse. This lasted about two months.

During the third month, I slowly began to be able to make it outside. I would walk about ten meters outside, and that would be my limit. I would sometimes attempt to walk to the milk bar and back (about 100 meters down the street); some days, I could only make it halfway and would have to turn back and go back to bed. Every day or two, though, I slowly walked farther and farther. After the third month, my energy was back to about 60 percent.

As the doctor told me that I would be fine after recovering from the Glandular Fever, I thought that I could start pushing myself slowly again. As I was feeling better again (about 60 percent better), I went back to work full time again. I worked as a personal trainer and taught dance classes. I have never been unfit in my life, so as I still felt 60 percent up to par,I I just thought that it was a sign of me losing some fitness after having been sick and without exercise for three months. I began lifting weights in the gym again. Before I got sick, I had been easily able to go for one intense hour with the weights. To me, there was no better feeling than smashing myself in the gym and leaving feeling like I'd just had an amazing workout. As I had taken three months off from being sick, and I felt still unwell (despite the doctor's insistence that I should be fine by then), I found that I was only able to continue with the weights for about 10 minutes, and that was all I could do. I still felt very weak, and every time I lifted weights, I would get dizzy. I pushed through it, though, as I thought I was just suffering from being unfit.

I had a good period from January to February. Although I still felt a little unwell, I didn't really think anything of it. My Mum told me I had to take six months off of work – six months of totally resting. As the doctor told me differently and said I would start to feel better after a few weeks, I ended up going back to work anyway. I taught dance classes again, and every single time I taught them, I would get extremely dizzy. You know the feeling when you have just had half a bottle of alcohol at once? I'm talking about that kind of dizzy feeling – the kind where you just want to pass out. Silly me, though, kept dancing, thinking I was fit and healthy and that I wasn't going to let anything keep me down.

The last day of January, 2011, was the last day that I thought I was still re-gaining my health. I trained about four personal training clients that morning, and then we went out for breakfast. We had a paint balling game outside for two hours in 30 degree heat. By the end of the game, I started to feel unwell and dizzy again, but as my health had been steadily improving, I didn't think too much of it. I had to sleep in the car before leaving, and I got the feeling through my body just like I did when I'd had glandular fever – one of those" uh oh" moment. I slept and felt okay again, so we went into the city and up to the Eureka sky deck, Melbourne's tallest building. The adrenaline kicked in (I'm terrified of heights.), and I really felt alive! Afterward, we ate delicious wraps and went to get some ice cream. As I was eating the ice cream and enjoying a great day, I got that "uh oh, here we go again" feeling and became very exhausted. It wasn't just a tired feeling where you feel a little sleepy and like you need a coffee or a nap. It was a feeling that came with extreme bodily fatigue, weakness, and dizziness, and a overall sense of illness. This event marked the beginning of my 2.5 year journey with Chronic Fatigue. After a few days of feeling horrible, I went in to see a different doctor. I told him what had been going on, and he said, "Alan you have chronic fatigue syndrome." I got some more blood tests done, and in about a week, I saw him again. I sat down in his exam room, and he asked, " Alan, what can I do for you?"

I told him, "Well, I have Chronic Fatigue Syndrome, as you said..." He immediately denied ever saying that and informed me that he would never say that to me. I told him several times that he in fact did say it to me, and I told him word for word what he had said to me, but he still denied saying it. It was like he was afraid to work with me, mainly because it was too complicated of a disease to treat.

I had CAT scans done on my brain to determine the cause of the dizziness. In fact, I had scans done all over my body.

I even had a test performed in which I ran on a treadmill while they measured my vital signs.

After the tests, I saw another doctor who was suppose to specialize in helping CFS sufferers. He put me on vitamin D drops and Q 10 tablets and scheduled me for more expensive tests.

I saw a neurologist who told me nothing and charged $450 for six minutes with him.

I went to a dizzy-day clinic that also charged me a bit to perform the same few tests that the neurologist had done.

All of my blood work was still coming back as normal, but I didn't want to give up hope of finding a diagnosis.

I then saw a CFS specialist in Melbourne. He was suppose to be one of the best in Australia. I went with my mum as she wanted to know what was going on. He said the same things as other doctors that there was not much he can do. He did however tried to get me to sign up for weekly injections of vitamin c, vitamin b and glutathione. I know all about the supplements as I have done a lot of study trying to get myself better. The injections seemed to be a good idea, however when I asked how much he replied;

"$200 each per injection. You would need to have them 3 times a week here for a total of 8 weeks. "

He also said it might work or might not but was worth a try

I told my mum NO!! I am not paying $1800 per week for 8 weeks for something that may or may not work.

Once again, I told my mum it's just another doctor/specialist that wants peoples money.

The visit was $450 and I was no better off.

I saw another doctor who told me that anti-depressants would help with my fatigue and dizziness. I didn't want to go on them, as I hate taking stuff I am unsure of the science behind those types of drugs, but he said they would help lessen the fatigue and dizziness, and at that point, I was willing to try anything. He also suggested sleeping tablets and explained that lack of sleep was a likely explanation for my being so tired all of the time. "If you don't have a good night's sleep," he explained, "of course your going to be tired in the morning." I tried to explain to him that my situation was a different kind of tired, but once again, he didn't believe me and said to take the sleeping tablets, so I took them.

I must admit that the first few weeks were awesome. I would take the sleeping tablet, and within two minutes, I would basically fall asleep on the table or on the couch. I felt really, really groggy but it was a great feeling, because I knew I was going to be able to go to sleep fast. Hooray!! My celebration was short-lived, however; the sleeping tablets worked for getting me to bed, but I would wake up around 2am and be wide awake. About two or three weeks later, the effect wore off, but I couldn't go to bed without them. So, to get to sleep, I then started taking 1.5 tablets. Another two weeks passed, and I increased the dosage to two tablets. I knew I shouldn't be taking them in a higher quantity than prescribed, but I needed them to get to sleep. I was on two tablets per night for about four months. I went to the doctor every week, and every two weeks, he would change my sleeping tablet. Some were slow release (so I would get better sleep during the night), and some were fast acting (so I would go to sleep straight away). I was now hooked on sleeping tablets, and my fatigue wasn't getting any better, as the doctors had said that it would.

At one point, I took a special sleeping tablet from the doctor that was supposed to be the best sleeping medication on the market. That night, I stayed up having hallucinations. I had the worst anxiety I had ever experienced, and I couldn't breathe properly. For some reason, I just couldn't catch my breath, and I was really panicky. When I laid down, I kept feeling people on my bed, pulling at my bed sheets, and on top of me yelling at me. It was the scariest thing ever!! Every time I tried to go to sleep, within one minute, I would hear whispering in my ear, and I would feel like people were in my room, coming to get me. It was horrible. It was like a nightmare coming to life. I saw the doctor the following night, and he said that such a reaction had never happened before, so he booked me an appointment with a psychiatrist.

$420 later, I left, once again feeling really let down and that people just wanted my money. I explained to the psychiatrist that I had been diagnosed with Chronic Fatigue Syndrome, and I told him about the episode I'd had with the hallucinations while taking the new sleeping tablet. He said, " That would never happen, and in my 20 years of experience, this is the first time I have ever heard of someone experiencing hallucinations from a sleeping tablet." As soon as he said that, I instantly thought, "What a shit talker!"

I told him I didn't believe in the supernatural and that I am a very logical person, so it would have to be the sleeping tablet. He didn't believe me and kept asking me strange questions. Here is a conversation we had once:

DOC: " I don't care if you don't believe in the supernatural; were they real?"

ME :" Well, they weren't real, because there is no such thing, so no."

DOC: " But were they real to you?"

ME: "No, they were from the sleeping tablet. It must have done something to my brain."

DOC: "Well, in my 20 years of experience, this has never happened, so I am thinking you did really have people in your room."

ME: "Ummmm...No, it was from the sleeping tablet."

Basically, it went back and forth, and he kept thinking I was lying to him. It is really funny how I all of a sudden tried a new sleeping tablet, and that very night, I had hallucinations. It doesn't take a genius to work out that it was the tablet affecting my brain. I went back to my old sleeping tablet, and I had an okay night again. I told the psychiatrist I had seen so many different people about my fatigue that wont go away, and that that was one of the reasons why I was seeing him. He wrote a letter to my doctor saying that he suspected I was suffering from "moderate depression."

At this point, I began to feel really pissed off. All of these medical professionals just seemed to have no idea what they were doing. I would say a good 90 percent of people suffering from CFS have gone through the same thing. You have seen 10-50 different people, and they all think you're depressed when you aren't. Then, you just get frustrated because you know you're not depressed. Depression and chronic fatigue are two completely different things.

I wake up every morning wanting to go for a run, go to the gym, and lift weights. I want to work full time. I want to go out and enjoy the sun. I want to have a few drinks and a laugh with friends. I want to drive down to see my family on the weekends. I have a to-do list with over 200 things I want to do, but I wake up in the morning feeling so sick and fatigued that all I can do is lay in bed. I eventually came to the conclusion that everyone in the health field was dumb and had no idea how to help me. I realized two years later that I had to do everything myself and learn as much as I could about this disease on my own, in order to get any helpful results.

I have researched my illness every single day from the beginning. As soon as I first got sick, I began was Googling "glandular fever" and learning what everyone had to say. In 2.5 years of having chronic fatigue, I have read and heard almost every single thing there is to know about so-called cures and treatments for CFS, many from companies just trying to rip people off. I have over $3000 worth of supplements that I have bought. (I will include the photo for everyone to see.) When you try and try to do everything you can to help yourself, but nothing seems to work, you begin to feel hopeless and that nothing will ever help you to feel better. Your latest research will lead you to another supplement, which claims that it cures or helps with fatigue and CFS; there will be raving reviews stating that it's a new miracle supplement/herb that has helped thousands of people. I will often do my research, buy a supplement, and almost always think, "Wow! Another waste of $60!"

I have tried many different diets, as well. I would say I have tried at least ten of them, ranging from cutting out dairy and gluten to going on a total detox and sticking to a strict program from the naturopath for about four months. When I didn't feel any better in four months,I I thought, "What's the use?" I then went back to eating my comfort foods and drinking my coffee and didn't feel any worse off. The only difference is that, if you eat junk foods while suffering from CFS, you're going to put on weight more quickly, because you're not exercising, so you really have to be careful with eating crap foods. I went from having a six pack and a muscular body to being very unhappy with my body. Being a fitness junkie, I have never really had a unhealthy figure before. So, because me being unhappy with my body and unable to exercise, I really have to be careful what I eat. Otherwise, I would have to apply for the next Santa Clause job!

Living with Chronic Fatigue Syndrome for almost three years was such a mind battle. Nothing I did seemed to make it better. For most people, all they need is a good sleep, and they feel good the next day. It wouldn't have mattered if I'd had 10-20 hours sleep. I would still wake up just as fatigued as if I hadn't slept at all. Do you remember that feeling when you were in high school or uni, and you were up until 3am trying to complete your assignments or cram for a test? Remember how tired you were? Imagine feeling ten times worse than that every single day. Imagine feeling like that at night time, sleeping for nine hours, waking up, and still feeling like that. Imagine what it would be like to go through it for just one week. You would go nuts, right? I had to deal with it for almost three years, and there are plenty of people who have had it a lot longer than I have. There were times when I wanted to give in. It just got to be too much for me. As I was repeatedly let down by my friends, I thought I could never open up to anyone else and ask for help, as I felt that I was constantly bothering people. Often, I thought about what it would be like if I just killed myself, but the thought of my mum, girlfriend, and best friend being sad made me realize that was never an option. I knew I had to just go through it, even if it meant I was basically a cripple for the rest of my life. I often thought about what would happen if it just went away completely. For instance, what if i woke up in the morning, and it had just gone away? Unfortunately, that never happen. I even thought that maybe this was all a nightmare, and I would wake up and feel better soon. Sadly enough, it was real, and it was something I had to go through daily. I struggled every day to wake up, and sometimes, I would stay in bed all day. On other days, I would get out of bed and eat breakfast. As soon as I'd had breakfast, I would have to go back to bed. The fatigue was unbearable, and I felt like I had been awake for six days straight. Two years went by, and it was still the same, so I knew I had to do something about it.

I started trying to stay awake out of bed for as long as possible. It was a nightmare! I could only stay out of bed for ten minutes, and then the fatigue got so bad that I would get that deathly feeling, and it just felt like my immune system was eating itself. As soon as that feeling would come, all I could do was go to bed. It used to happen all the time, and several times, I just collapsed from mere exhaustion. I literally had no energy left in my body to stand up or even talk.

I kept working at it, and soon, ten minutes had become 20 minutes, and so on. By about 2-3 months, I was out of bed for the majority of the day. This greatly improved my quality of sleep. With Chronic Fatigue Syndrome, most people have insomnia on top of it. Too much resting and sleeping during the day results in not being able to sleep at night, so I made a massive effort to reset my body's internal clock. I did anything it took to stay out of bed. This did help me sleep better at night, but it was a slow process to recovery.

Better quality sleep= faster recovery. Sleep gives your body a better chance to rest and heal overnight.

I tried all the diets under the sun, and I am sure you have, too, if you suffer from CFS. Any diet or eating plan I tried didn't make me feel better. I will cut to the chase and say that the only diet that has worked is the one I am on now, and I plan to be on it for a very long time. I cut out anything that was artificial or processed. I would say that my diet consists of 80% natural products, meaning I only eat stuff that is grown or raised, such as vegetables, fruits, seeds, lean meats, fish, and nuts. Nutrition is a massive part of getting better, and there's not a single miracle diet that will work for everyone. For example, some people are sensitive to gluten, and some people aren't.

What I would suggest is doing an elimination diet to start off with, so you know what your body likes and what it doesn't.

This basically means that you're only allowed to eat certain foods for a small period of time, and then you slowly introduce different foods into your diet. For instance, if you cut dairy out of your diet completely for 3-4 weeks, you might have one glass of milk three times a day after those weeks of abstaining from it, in order to test how your body will react. If your symptoms are worse that day, or the next couple of days, you know that you shouldn't be consuming dairy products. You keep doing this until everything is eliminated, and then you will know what your body likes and what it doesn't like. You need to feed your body stuff it likes. I don't mean the tastes either. "Likes" means the foods your body needs to heal itself.

Foods to Include in your Elimination Diet:

All fresh fruit, excluding citrus fruits (oranges, grapefruits, limes, and lemons)

All fresh vegetables, excluding tomatoes, eggplants, or potatoes.

You can eat rice, but don't eat any wheat, corn, barley, spelt, oats, or anything that contains gluten.

No legumes are allowed (soybeans, soy milk, beans, peas, lentils, or oats).

No nuts or seeds are allowed.

Only eat fish, turkey, or lamb; no other meats are allowed.

Cut out dairy products; only almond, rice, or coconut milks are allowed as replacements

Only allowed pressed olive oil, flaxseed oil, or coconut oil for cooking.

Only fresh water is allowed. Try to filter it, if you can. You are allowed some herbal teas, as long as they are organic and don't have any other chemicals in them.

You are allowed to have any herb added to your food, but you are not allowed any sauces you buy from the supermarket, like tomato sauce (ketchup), mustard, soy sauce, vinegar, etc.

No sweeteners are to be added to your elimination diet. You are allowed Stevia if you must have something, but it's best if you don't have it either.

Now you know what you can eat. You can eat anything you want, as long as its on the list. You don't have to count calories; you can eat as much as you want. Make sure to drink plenty of filtered water. You can buy filtered jugs for very cheap. If you have the money, go buy one of them now.

You're going to be on the elimination diet for about 3-4 weeks. You will then slowly start reintroducing foods that you weren't allowing yourself to eat. You might start with the milk and have a glass of milk in the morning, a glass at lunch, and for a glass with dinner or when you go to bed. Monitor your symptoms. If you have no symptoms for the next couple of days, then reintroduce something else. If you introduce a certain food that your body reacts to, you know to cut it out of your diet.

The reaction from the food could be anything that makes your problems with sleep, mood, energy, and digestion, or your cold-like symptoms worse.

Also, reintroducing the foods could make your CFS symptoms worse, too. You need to watch out for this. Keep a notebook handy, and write down everything that goes into your mouth and what your symptoms are over the next couple of days. By about a month's time, you should know exactly what your body can handle and what it cannot.

Most people don't understand what Chronic Fatigue Syndrome is. I once new a girl who had glandular fever and she had to take 6 months off school. I saw that she was always on Facebook and updating her status about watching movies in bed. I kept thinking that the only reason she was tired was because she was always in bed. I thought that she was just lazy, as I was comparing the amount of energy she seemed to have to the amount that I had. People can tell you all of their different symptoms, but because you don't experience them yourself, you have no idea what they are going through. Everyone gets headaches or has gotten a headache at least once in their lives, so when someone says he has a headache, we all have a general idea of what it's like. You can't say the same about bowel cancer, AIDS, being blind, or having CFS, for example. It's something that not everyone will understand, because they haven't been through it themselves. As I have already mentioned, CFS an illness that is so bad that I would rather be in pain. It's like you have the flu, but multiply the intensity by ten. You can feel your immune system and every cell in your body eating you alive. It feels like every cell in your body is dying. I felt like I was dead, and it was the most horrible thing I could ever imagine. I often think about when I had my legs operated on when I was about 17 years old, because I had Compartment Syndrome, in which the muscle gets too big for the fascia. I had nerve damage from dancing on it like this for too long. After the surgery, one of my legs got infected. I remember lying down in bed, and if I moved my leg even one centimeter, I would scream. The pain was unbearable. A few times, I was in so much pain that I passed out in bed. No pain killers (even the ones from the hospital) made it better. Now, if I had the choice between being in massive amounts of pain like I was then, or to have CFS when it's really bad, I seriously wouldn't know which one is better or worse. At least the pain improved after three months, so I would probably choose the pain over the fatigue.

When you say to people that you are fatigued, they just think that you're tired. Then, when you say to them, "No, I'm not tired. I'm fatigued," then they look at you as if you are crazy. You have to explain to them that being tired means that you want to sleep, and you can sleep, while being fatigued means that you want to sleep but you can't.

The fatigue is so bad that it keeps you awake. It would be similar to having a bad migraine at night time. That would keep you up, as it would just be throbbing all night. Imagine if there weren't any painkillers to make it go away, and you just had to deal with that the pain.

Before I got sick, I used to love life so much! I was always that person that had more energy then everyone else. I was working 105 hours a week for about a year, so you can imagine how much energy I used to have. I was just high on life. I loved my life; I loved being alive; I loved my friends, music, the summer, having coffee, having a laugh; I loved basically everything. I was working so much because I loved helping people. I even trained people every morning from 6am to 9am, Monday to Friday, for free. There were many days when I would wake up and go to work, only to realize that no one had shown up for that day. But, that was fine by me! I got more and more tired as time went on, but I never thought that I would get sick. I had heard of chronic fatigue before but never knew it could be that bad. I thought you just got tired a lot, and my thought process was, "Well, you just need to get some sleep, and you'll be okay." If I knew back then what I know now, I would have only worked about 40 hours a week, not trained for free, resisted working from home so often, and realized that having five coffees a day wasn't healthy for me. I wish I had eaten better, slept about 2-3 hours a night longer, and taken the weekends off to enjoy and relax and have a good time.

There is no magic pill for anything in life, so once you have some illness, you can either feel depressed and ask, "What if I had done this differently?" or you can realize that you have something to deal with now, and it's up to you to change it so that you can get better.

My advice with anyone suffering from chronic fatigue is that you need to look at what you're doing.

How many hours per week do you work?

How many coffees do you need during the day?

How many hours of sleep do you get?

Do you eat healthily?

What do you think eating healthily means?

Do you smoke or drink?

Are you stressed?

You need to understand that your health is number one. Nothing else matters if you don't have you health. You need your health to be happy and function day by day.

For everyone who has CFS, you now have a greater understanding of what you can do to get better.

Take the bad experience, and turn it into a good one. Think positively, and know that you're going to get better one day. It will probably not happen overnight, but it might happen in a few weeks, a few months, etc. In fact, depending on how bad it is and whats going on inside your body, it could take many years to recover. What I am saying is that you have the tools to recover more quickly, and you now know what you can do and what you can't. Use your mindset to overcome this illness, and understand that you will get better. You are not the only one suffering; there are millions and millions of people all over the world who have CFS. Use all the information you have read about and learned about to your advantage, and I hope you have a much faster recovery to better health.

Chapter 13: The History Of The Fruitarian Diet

Most people are not aware of the long history of people having huge success on a Fruit based diet. Anne Osborne wrote about this in an article for the UK Fruitfest newsletter:

A Recent History of the Fruitarian Diet **by Anne Osborne**

Being part of today's growing raw vegan community, has given me an interest in looking at our fruity roots and those who went before us; in this article, I will examine the recent history of the fruitarian diet and look at some of the pioneers who by their research, experiences, and enthusiasm helped to bring this way of living to fruition in the lives of many.

Although, I believe thousands of years ago, we were happy and healthy little fruit eaters living on an edenic fruitarian diet in a forest environment; this article will focus on the history of the fruit diet over the last two centuries.

To understand the recent beginnings of the fruit diet, I think we need to first examine the ideas of the Natural Hygiene Movement, which started in the 1820's and 1830's in Europe and the United States.

Those interested in Natural Hygiene believed that it was the human body alone that healed from a state of illness and it was not any allopathic, herbal, or homeopathic remedies that cured sickness.

However, for the body to heal quickly and effectively, it needed certain conditions, these included fresh air, an adequate level of exercise, an appropriate amount of sleep, a pure water supply, and a natural diet.

This then opened up a whole can of Tomatoes, namely, what then is a 'natural' food for humans? In order for a foodstuff to qualify, it needed to satisfy certain criteria:

It had to be a food that humans found delicious in its totally unprocessed state, that is fare that was appetising without cooking, mixing, or changing it in any way from its natural form.

Then the food needed to be easily digested by humans. It is no good how delicious we may find a food to be if our bodies cannot digest it efficiently in its natural raw state.

And thirdly, it needed to be a food that could supply us with all the macro and micro nutrients we require to thrive and live healthy and happy lives. No matter how tasty a food may be, or how wonderfully it digests; if we cannot obtain our daily nutritional needs from it, then it cannot be our ideal fodder!

Fruit can certainly fulfil all three of these

criteria, and so it came about that in these early days of the Natural Hygiene Movement, authors and researchers started to promote fruit as being a perfect food for human beings. One of the earliest of the modern researchers was a European called Gustav Schlickeysen; Schlickeysen spent much time researching human physiology and anatomy, the results of his studies were published in his 1877 book, 'Fruit and Bread'.

This work contains his Comparative Analysis Tables, the first of their kind I have found, but subsequently much copied in natural diet and vegetarian books. The tables can be useful for arranging data in a way that allows for easy comparison of the anatomical features of different groups of animals.

By comparing human anatomy with the other mammals, Schlickeysen concluded that, by design, humans are very much fruit eaters; and in every way, our anatomy compares most strongly to the frugivorous Anthropoid Apes.

Our teeth, our intestines, our placentas, and our eyes match most closely with our simian cousins. Schlickeysen also advocated whole unprocessed grains in addition to the juicy fruits.

His ideas would have been very radical for his time and Schlickeysen does indeed seem to be a pioneer in showing that the frugivorous diet was best suited to humans and that their anatomy was that of a fruit eater.

Schlickeysen says on page 111 of **'Fruit and Bread'**:

"Take for example, a man who lives in the free air and in daily communication with Nature, who enjoys the blessings of willing labor, who eats the juicy fruits of the garden , and drinks from the pure fountain, whose eye is clear and whose cheek is crimsoned by the blessed sunlight, and compare him with the one who lives in the foul air of some great factory and who subsists on flesh, and potatoes, beer and coffee. Look only at two such men standing as the representatives of two distinct systems of diet and life, and say which system is to be preferred."

At no point in his book, did Schlickeysen use the term 'fruitarian', but rather

fruit diet'.

However, Schlickeysen's peer, Emmet Densmore does use the word 'fruitarian', in his 1892 book: 'How Nature Cures and the Natural Food of Man'; so it would seem the word came into use sometime after 1877 but before 1892.

Emmet was another of the pioneers of the fruit-based diet.

However, unlike Schlickeysen, Emmet did not advocate grains believing them to contain matter which silted up and aged the human body.

But he believed that fruit was a perfect food for humans because it contained the least 'earthy matter' of any foodstuff. Emmet was influenced in his ideas by a British doctor, Charles de Lacy Evans, who had also done a lot of research into fruit based diets and had written a book about his findings.

De Lacy Evans' book, published in 1879, was entitled 'How to Prolong Life' ; in this work, De Lacy Evans described in detail how the 'earthy matter' in foods negatively affected the body and caused aging and degeneration.

Fruit was advocated by De Lacy Evans as the most appropriate food for humans because it contained the least 'earthy matter' whilst containing all the nutrients humans needed to thrive.

In his book, on page 79 he says:

"We see that fruits, as distinct from vegetables, have the least amount of earthy salts."

And on page 82:

"it has been argued that fruits will not sustain life because they do not contain sufficient nitrogen; this argument is founded upon a theory which is demonstrably incorrect, and it is an ascertained fact that fruit alone will support life in good bodily health."

Subsequent advocates of a fruit diet who were influenced by De Lacy Evans' theory included Hereward Carrington, and the mid Twentieth Century health author Hilton Hotema.

Then, towards the end of the 19th Century, saw the emergence of one of the most influential pioneers of the fruitarian diet; his name was Arnold Ehret, born in Baden, in Germany in 1866.

After suffering serious health issues in his early years, Ehret discovered the benefits of fasting and the fruit diet, which allowed his body to regain a high level of health and wellness.

He states in his book, **"Rational Fasting"**, on page 12:

"After a two year strict fruit diet, with calculated fasting cures, I had attained a degree of health which is simply not imaginable nowadays."

Ehret also believed that exercise was a vital component of a healthy lifestyle and he combined exercise with dietary recommendations for his clients.

Ehret emigrated to the United States in 1914, where he opened a sanatorium in Alhambra, California, and he also travelled to other cities , giving lectures.

Another German-born pioneer of the fruit diet was the medical doctor O.L.M. Abramowski; born in 1852, Abramowski emigrated to Australia in1884.

After turning his health around, from being near death's door to having abundant energy and vibrant health, by adopting a fruit diet, Abramowski was keen to save more lives.

He did this by providing a fruitarian diet to his patients at his Mildura hospital in Victoria, Australia.

This was one of the first fruitarian hospitals, of recent times. Abramowski got such great results with his patients, that many of his nurses adopted the fruit diet too!

During the typhoid epidemic from 1903-1908, the death rate in nearby hospitals was 13%, but in Abramowski's establishment, the death rate was only 1%!

I feel very grateful for these innovators and health enthusiasts who spent many years, and expended much energy, to help people heal, whilst also documenting their discoveries and successes; they have helped pave the way for all those of us who follow in their fruity footsteps.

Chapter 14: What Aggravates Pain?

Several studies and researches have been conducted, but until now, researchers are still clueless as to the things that aggravate pain. It was discovered, however, that the things which can alleviate pain are also the same things that can aggravate it. Furthermore, according to their studies, people generally do not know what exactly are the things or factors that can alleviate or aggravate their pain. Here are several factors:

Activity can aggravate the pain and worsen the situation. For example, a person who sprained his ankle is not allowed to move freely without a cane or support. If he uses his feet without support, the sprained ankle will have to carry the full weight thus, applying pressure on the injured ankle will make it worse and walking will be more painful. Changing positions can also aggravate pain because it adds pressure and force on the injured area.

Eating is sometimes helpful, but oftentimes, it aggravates pain as well. When the person is sick, it is best to give him soft foods like mashed potatoes or porridge. In some situations however, even soft foods are still painful. Just the act of opening the mouth is already painful in some situations. Chewing is not advisable for tooth aches and during post dental surgeries. Intake of acidic foods and liquids is also prohibited, especially in the case of ulcer and canker sores. Kissing or talking is equally painful when the lip is busted or when there's a wound in the mouth. Furthermore, certain foods can cause adverse reactions in the body. For example, acidic type foods can exasperate arthritis symptoms. Gluten and milk products are known to elevate symptoms in the body causing inflammation.

As much as activity aggravates pain, inactivity can also aggravate it. Inactivity causes blood circulation to be stagnant and it produces pain. It produces a numbing pain when you sit for long period of time. If you are hospitalized and your position is unchanged for several days, you will develop bed sores and it's painful.

Stress also is a contributing factor that aggravates pain. Stress is known to be the "silent killer." When the body perceives a threat, it enters into a "fight or flight" response. When we are prepared to "fight", the adrenaline in our body increases and the cortisol hormone rises. This is normal and usually drops off when the stress is dealt with. However, if a person is in constant stress and has an overexposure to cortisol in the body, their health is quick to deteriorate and the body's healing process is ruptured. Sleeplessness also impedes the immune system from working properly thus, inflammation and swelling becomes worse. A fresh wound can also start to bleed and may reopen if a person is emotionally unstable, angry, or depressed.

As much as medical treatment can alleviate and relieve pain altogether, it can also make it worse. There are medications which produce harmful and painful side effects to the person being treated. For example, aspirins; they are indeed pain relievers and very powerful at that, however, when taken on a daily basis, it destroys gastrointestinal lining causing painful spasms and acute pain in the stomach. Chemotherapy is also another factor which aggravates pain, as well as surgery.

In severe physical injuries, pressure is needed to stop the bleeding. There are times however, when touching the injured area is not very advisable. This is true with those injured in motor or vehicular accidents. One wrong touch on the affected area can kill the person or worsen the injury. There may be broken bones which are better left untouched and without pressure. Similarly, if the affected area is already infected and swelling is really severe, touching it becomes unbearably painful. This is the case of burn victims. The skin or the flesh is open and touching it is ultimately the most painful thing that they will hope never to experience. Antiseptic or cleaning their wound will make them cry in pain that is incomparable to anything else.

Temperature can also aggravate the pain. This is most often the case for older people. Arthritis and other joint problems are at their most painful during the winter season. Bone cancer patients are most susceptible to severe pain during the cold season. Skin problems on the other hand, are most painful during the hot season or summer when the skin becomes dry. This is most particularly true when perspiration seeps into the wound.

Poor posture can also exasperate the pain, especially for people who suffer back and neck pain. Slouching, sitting too long, standing with one hip jutting out, twisting the body, improper lifting, crossing legs, or caring a backpack on one shoulder are many of the ways that our bodies can be thrown out of alignment. It is important to get up and stretch when sitting in a chair or car for too long. Every couple hours is recommended. When watching television, face the screen head on rather than twisting your body to view the screen. Practice sitting up right when at the computer or using electronic devises. It is best to not keep your head in the down position for too long. Movement is the key to keeping muscles loose in the body.

environmental toxins can contribute to inflammation in the body and elevate the chronic pain. Toxins can include air quality, heavy metals in food or materials, pesticides, chemical fertilizers, antibiotics and hormones in food products, genetically modified foods, plastic containers, and nitrates in deli meats, artificial coloring/flavors/sweeteners, and chemical detergents. The list is endless. Eliminating or reducing these toxins in your environment is crucial. People even go another step further and partake in routine detoxes and cleanses to rid the body of these harmful toxins.

Chapter 15: Relax

If you are exhausted and tired all the time, it makes sense to step take a step back and relax. Here are the things that you can do to help you relax, enjoy life, and increase your energy:

Rest when you have to.

Do not push yourself too hard. Remember that it is important to rest from time to time.

Take some time off from work.

This is one of the most difficult, since we need to make a living and we have demands and tasks that need to be done. However, taking a little time off can help you gain clarity. We often are "too close to the situation" an get stressed over details of work. Taking some well deserved time off, even a few hours or days, can help you focus on what is really important so you can concentrate your efforts and be more effective.

Do repetitive motions.

Studies show that doing repetitive motions such as brushing your hair, knitting, or washing the dishes can actually help you relax.

Take time to be alone.

Being alone from time to time will help you relax. It aids in effectively dealing with personal issues that have been draining your energy.

Get organized.

If you want to avoid stress and increase your energy, then you have to organize your things. Organizing your personal and work space will help relax your mind and your body.

Smell the flowers.

Aromatherapy can help restore the balance in your body. It can also help you fight stress and anxiety.

Cuddle with your pet.

If you are feeling tired or exhausted, cuddling with your pet will instantly make you feel good. It will energize you and lift your spirit.

Have fun.

Go out and have fun! Having fun will help restore your energy. It will also keep you balanced while also relieving stress, depression, and anxiety. Here are the fun things that you can try:

- Go to a theme park.
- Go to a Karaoke bar and belt out some songs with your friends.
- Try something different like jet-skiing, bungee jumping, and hiking.
- Take up a new hobby

Tend to yourself.

It is best to tend to yourself and take care of your needs. A little "me time" works wonders.

Get enough sleep.

If you want to live a high energy life, getting good, quality sleep is a must. It is recommended that adults get from 7 to 9 hours daily. It is also best to have a fixed sleeping time to stablize your body clock. Avoid drinking coffee hours before your bedtime. It is also best to have a bedtime routine like taking a bath or reading inspirational quotes before sleeping. Take cat-naps.

Naps help restore your energy after a long day at work. It can improve your cognitive function and increase your energy throughout the day.

Focus on the present moment.

Do not dwell so much on the past or worry too much about the future. If you want to live a high-energy life, you have to focus on the present moment. You can do this by practicing mindfulness.

Take a breather.

When work seems hard and stressful, take time to take deep breaths. Go out of the office and take a five minute walk. This will help restore your energy and clear your head.

When you take time to relax, you will keep yourself balanced. You will increase your energy and vitality. When you find time to relax, you get to deal with the symptoms of chronic fatigue and exhaustion head on.

Chapter 16: Living Strong With Hypothyroidism

The thyroid gland responsible for producing thyroid hormones plays an important role in keeping your energy and metabolism in check. It's responsible for the proper functionality of your body, thus with a reduction in the thyroid hormones, your body overtime will face numerous problems.

Even though hypothyroidism is a lifelong condition, you don't have to be its victim, you don't have to suffer continuously from exhaustion, pain and all the numerous discomforts that accompany hypothyroidism. You can heal yourself naturally and even reverse hypothyroidism with your dedication and determination.

And let me clarify again, you can heal yourself completely through natural methods which means there's no surgeries or medications involved. All you need to do is bring some lifestyle and diet changes.

However, if you believe your doctor's prescribed medications or your current treatment will help you then you can follow that too along with the natural healing methods. You can use these natural healing techniques on the side to boost your overall healing process. These strategies will help to control your hypothyroidism all the while reversing your condition.

Natural effective methods to cure hypothyroidism

Adding maca root powder to your daily meals can greatly help with hypothyroidism. It's known to balance the hormones in the body and if you have observed in the previous chapters, hypothyroidism is nothing but a hormonal imbalance in the body. Hence, adding a scoop of maca powder to your smoothies or drinks daily could work wonders.

Try to steer clear of the chemicals fluoride and chloride as they are known to interfere with thyroid functions. You may need to filter your drinking water, even shower water, public pools and toothpastes that contain fluoride to help your condition.

Many patients who have stopped using plastic bottles and plastic containers reported that they faced lesser symptoms of hypothyroidism. The science behind it is the fact that plastics when exposed to high heat release chemicals at an accelerated rate which can wreak havoc on your hormone levels. Hence, it's advised to not use plastic containers to microwave food or store water in plastic bottles for long period of times.

Eliminate all nonstick cookware if you want to regain your health. Nonstick cookware might be handy to use but in the long run it causes more harm to health than good. Nonstick surfaces are usually made using harmful chemicals which not only lead to hormone disruption but also infertility and other health risks.

Coconut oil is known to have medium chain fatty acids that help improve thyroid functioning. Moreover, it naturally boosts energy and metabolism in the body. Coconut oil also actively raises the basal body temperature which helps patients with hypothyroidism. Thus, many use coconut oil in their daily meals to improve their thyroid functioning. You can use it as cooking oil or simply add it to milk or smoothies daily.

Another effective method is including kelp in your diet. Since patients with hypothyroidism have iodine deficiency, kelp (which have abundant iodine and other useful minerals for the body) can greatly help. However, patients with auto immune thyroid problems are not advised to take kelp as it's known to worsen the conditions further. In any case, discuss with your doctor before including kelp in your diet.

Consuming apple cider vinegar with honey daily can prove to be beneficial for you. Apple cider vinegar aids in detoxification and restore acid alkaline balance in the body. It helps to regulate hormonal imbalance and also helps in weight loss. Overall, consuming it on a regular basis will help improve your metabolism. Apple cider vinegar is not only useful for patients with hypothyroidism but also great for diabetic patients or individuals with high cholesterol or blood pressure.

Many also swear by fish oil supplements. Since fish oil contains abundance of omega 3 fatty acids, it helps fight inflammation and strengthens immunity. It effectively increases thyroid hormone uptake and maintains healthy functioning of your thyroid gland. If you are willing to include this method to your regimen make sure to check with your doctor first for the appropriate amount of dosage. Usually, doctors prescribe 3 gm per day but it can vary as well depending on the severity of your condition.

You may also use guggul to treat hypothyroidism. For those who are not familiar with Guggul, it's an herbal concoction that's made from the sap (gum resin) of the tree Commiphora Mukul. Years of research indicates that it's very effective in stimulating thyroid function. Moreover, it has anti-inflammatory properties. It also helps with weight loss and lowering cholesterol levels.

Usually 25 mg of guggul is prescribed per day but just to be on the safe side you should discuss with your doctor before deciding the dosage. Since guggul can interfere with estrogen, birth control pills or other medications, you should take your doctor's advice before consuming it. Also, when on guggul you should monitor your T3 and T4 levels often. Guggul actively stimulates conversion of T4 to T3.

Another great natural ingredient used in healing hypothyroidism is primrose oil. Evening primrose oil has abundant gamma linoleic acids (GLAs) which help to increase the levels of thyroid hormones in the body. Besides, it also help to cope with hair loss and heavy menstruation due to hypothyroidism.

Taking 200 to 100 mg of Siberian Ginseng can stimulate adrenal and thymus glands in your body. These two glands indirectly help to stimulate your thyroid gland. Hence, patients consume it twice daily to stimulate their thyroid functioning. Also, patients have reported that consuming this herb help alleviate fatigue, one of the most dreaded symptom of hypothyroidism.

Lifestyle changes

Curing your thyroid problem will not be easy and definitely will not occur within a flash. Thyroid problems arise after years and years of self-inducing poison. Much the same way, curing it is also a slow process and requires long term commitment. So, expect a year or so before you can heal yourself. If you are thinking that only including these natural methods will cure you then you are highly mistaken. Because relying on these natural herbs and supplements is only winning half the battle. One major part of healing yourself naturally involves some major changes in your lifestyle as well.

You can start with changing your sleeping pattern and waking up early in the morning every day. It might sound like an old and useless advice but you need the early morning sunlight to generate enough vitamin D in the body. Hypothyroidism is a result of deficiency of vitamin D. Hence, the simple act of waking up early and soaking up sunlight can work wonders in healing your body.

One major problem that hypothyroid patients face is the constant exhaustion. In order to deal with this problem you need to plan your meal throughout the day. Instead of having three major meals in a day, have a light breakfast and then get some mid lunch snacks. After lunch, have evening snacks too. The key here is to have moderate sized meals throughout the day so that your energy levels stay stable.

That said, I don't mean you can indulge in all kinds of fatty foods throughout the day. In order to cure this disease, you will have to be mindful of what you eat. Opt for whole foods and vegetables. You can never win this battle by relying on processed, fatty, junk foods. So, next time think twice before heating your convenient microwave meal. Like it or not but curing hypothyroidism will involve a lot of changes in your eating habits.

Next major change that you should bring in your lifestyle is physical activity. Exercise is an integral part of any healthy lifestyle but for hypothyroid patients exercise is even more important. You ask why? Simple. Patients with hypothyroidism easily gain weight even with an active lifestyle. This means hypothyroid patients will pile up on high levels of bad cholesterol if they remain completely sedentary. Hence, exercising daily is very important. Exercise will not only help you keep your waist size down but also increase your metabolism, give you a surge of energy and lower the bad cholesterol levels in the body.

You should also incorporate meditation and yoga in your daily life. Fighting with a disease can easily take its toll on even the strongest of persons. Sometimes you may need to distract yourself from the pressure and stress of living with hypothyroidism. Hence, you can try meditation to calm your mind and let yourself relax a bit.

Lastly, establish a sleep schedule. Pick a time and religiously go to bed at the same time every night. This will tell your internal clock that at this particular hour, it's time to hit the snooze. Hypothyroid patients suffer from fatigue throughout the day and therefore it's important for them to have enough sleep daily. Plus, fixing a specific time to go to bed makes it way easier to wake up in the morning. Train your body and you will see the results for yourself.

Exercises for hypothyroidism

If you have hypothyroidism, you already know how hard it can be to shed a few pounds. Even with limiting food intakes and an active lifestyle, your body constantly piles on the pounds. The reason? Your slowed metabolism and your high carb diet. We are a generation that heavily relies on carbohydrate. Starting from white bread to pasta to sugar, we love foods that have carbs in it.

The only problem with carbs is that the type of carbs we eat are often stripped of their nutrients. For instance, white rice or white bread are refined carbs that have little nutritional value compared to brown rice or brown bread. On top of that, refined carbs cause sugar spikes in the body that leave you hungry for more food. With all these on your plate, it can be tough to get rid of the bad cholesterol and pounds of fat in your body. Hence, doctors recommend at least 30 minutes of physical activity every day.

The best way to shed pounds is by doing 30 minutes of cardio. You don't even need equipment for this exercise. All you need is a pair of shoes and you are good to go. If you are fond of dancing, you can also opt for cardio dance workouts instead of the plain old running or walking.

Another good physical exercise for hypothyroidism is interval aerobic exercises. In this exercise you perform short burst of high intensity aerobic exercises and then let your body rest for a brief amount of time. For example, 5 minutes of aerobic exercise and then 30 seconds of resting time. You can choose any activity in this section, for instance, walking, running or bicycling etc.

Apart from cardio and aerobic exercises, strength training is also very important to help your body shed those extra pounds from hypothyroidism. Muscle building will help you in burning calories throughout the day all while increasing your body's metabolism. Hence, you should include some leg lunges, push-ups, squats, or overhead presses in your exercise routine.

Chapter 17: Muscle Fatigue

This is a condition in which the muscles of the body are unable to exert normal force, or an extra effort is required to achieve the desired amount of force. Muscle fatigue is due to exercise induced fatigue or genetic conditions leading to muscle weakness.

Exercised induced fatigue occurs when the body momentarily exhausts its supply of energy believed to result from disruptions in the flow of calcium through the muscles. It usually disappears after rest.

Muscle fatigue arises from the accumulation of lactic acid and is also associated with muscle soreness.

Muscle weakness can eventually lead to heart problems and breathing problems. Chronic conditions like Lou Gehrig's disease resulting from muscle weakness can cause death when the patient becomes slowly paralyzed and stops breathing. The processes in the muscles and nerve cells at the site of an area with fatigue largely contribute to the fatigue of that muscle. In addition, genetic and acquired conditions can lead to muscle fatigue.

Fatigue After Eating

Fatigue after eating is largely caused by stress and vitamin or mineral deficiencies. There should be no need to worry if you get an occasional fatigue after eating. It only becomes a problem if it occurs after every meal. This is an indicator that your body is not functioning well.

Symptoms:

Stomach pain.

Diarrhea.

Feeling bloated.

Nausea.

Loss of energy.

Lack of concentration.

Nervousness.

Vomiting.

Confusion.

Muscle weakness.

Sleepiness.

Decreased level of consciousness.

Nausea is the sensation that you need to vomit. When you feel bloated you feel the stomach is overstretched and filled with gas. Nervousness is a feeling of uneasiness.

Causes of Fatigue After Eating:

We previously cited that excessive sugar is a contributor to fatigue. It is important to note that foods contain sugars. Breakdown of these sugars take place fast but the energy obtained from them is not long-lasting. Hypoglycemia is also a major cause of fatigue after eating. Other causes of fatigue after eating are excessive sugars in food, stress, overeating, overstimulation, under stimulation, sleep deprivation, boredom, jetlag, and lack of exercise.

Medical Conditions That Cause Fatigue After Eating:

Kidney diseases

The kidney is tasked with excretion of toxins and unwanted materials from the blood. Kidney diseases make the kidney unable to effectively carry out this task. Accumulation of toxins in the body causes fatigue. If the kidney does not remove excess glucose cells will be unable to uptake that glucose causing fatigue like we discussed earlier.

Pregnancy

During early pregnancy, the body produces more of progesterone. This is responsible for making the woman feel sluggish and sleepy. In addition, the body produces more blood to transport nutrients to the unborn. This translates into more energy requirements for the heart and other organs. This strain on the energy to do other activities is felt as fatigue.

Allergies

Seasonal allergies are associated with sleep disturbances. The immune response characteristic of allergies requires energy to respond to otherwise non harmful objects in the body.

Insomnia and jetlag.

Insomnia is disorder in sleep initiation, maintenance, duration and quality of sleep. As such the body does not enjoy restorative effect of sleep. Jetlag is temporary sleep disorder in the body's circadian rhythm which is a disruption of internal body clock.

Parkinson's disease

Scientists suggest that fatigue in Parkinson's disease could be as a result of changes in the brain of the patient.

However, patients suffer from sleep disorders which could also be contributors to fatigue.

Muscular dystrophy

Muscular dystrophies occasion the weakening of the muscles of the body. As such the muscles decline in force and cannot sufficiently deliver enough energy to undertake some activities.

Heart diseases, autoimmune disease, anemia, fibromyalgia, depression and physical or mental trauma are other medical conditions that fatigue after eating. You can refer to other sections of this book that have discussed them in more details.

Chronic Fatigue Syndrome Symptoms

Sleep that does not make you feel refreshed.

Muscle pain.

Joint pain without swelling or redness.

Headaches of a new type of severity.

Sore throat that is frequent and recurring.

Chronic fatigue syndrome has no known conventional treatment. The complementary and alternative treatments are commonly used. An Asian herb called **Ginseng** is used to increase energy and fight fatigue. Nicotinamide Adenine Dinucleotide (NADH) is also used as treatment because it plays a crucial role of cellular energy production. **Dexedrine** is a stimulant that treats CFS.

Chapter 18: Methods Of Dealing With Chronic Stress

One common complaint in the field of stress management is the problem of putting the brakes on when stress occurs. The HPA axis gets activated in the presence of chronic stress conditions. After an extended period of exposure to stress, the epinephrine surges damage arteries and blood vessels increasing the risk of stroke and heart attack. Due to the elevated cortisol level, a series of physiological changes occur that help to replenish the energy used up during the stress response. But, one side effect is the formation of fat tissue that leads to weight gain. Cortisol not only increases appetite, but it also makes people put on weight. Here are some methods of dealing with the stress response.

Use of Relaxation Response

People can counter stress using a combination of responses that combine to induce relaxation. These techniques include a focus on soft words, deep breathing, yoga, prayer, tai chi, and thinking about calming scenes.

Controlling Blood Pressure with Relaxation Training☐

A study took place using a group of people undergoing hypertension. The research helps determine a realistic method of countering chronic stress. Though the results showed many methods they were not a cure-all, some of them were worth trying. In one instance, one half of a group of 120 people got training in relaxation response while the other group used information on control of blood pressure. After eight weeks, they noticed that more than half of the group that underwent relaxation response training showed a drop-in blood pressure. With continued medication, 50% of them were able to do without at least one of their blood pressure medications while 18% of the whole group was able to stop their blood pressure medication in its entirety.

Use of Physical Activity

People can withhold stress buildup by indulging in physical activity. Exercises of all kinds help, beginning with a brisk walk when one feels stressed to regular high-intensity workouts in the gym help one avoid stress. One of the best things that happens when you exercise is that you develop deep breathing. This helps soothe the nerves like the movement therapies that include qi gong, tai chi, and yoga among others. One develops mental focus and a calm mind.

Get Social Support

Co-workers, friends, family, spouses, and companions can combine to form that life-enhancing net which can help you reduce stress. It is the dissipation of emotional tensions that contributes the most to calming the mind. This can increase longevity in the long run but in the short-term perspective, it helps you improve the quality of your life. It ranges from timely support to good company at dinner. You will have the best advice to help you through those torrid times of chronic stress.

The Brain Immune System

Immune events remain controlled by the brain through exertions on the HPA axis. Vegetative functions such as appetite, growth, thyroid function, sleep, and reproduction remain controlled by the hypothalamus that occupies a small part of the diencephalon. It helps with adaptation through neural connections to the limbic system and involves the emotional and neuroendocrine responses in the face of stress.

"Emotional stress is often harder to identify. Things you thought you'd put behind you can be lurking inside, ready to resurface at any moment" (Pick, 2018).

How does this happen? Information from the periphery of the brain converges in the hypothalamus, the efferent link to the visceral brain. The information from the outer regions gets integrated with the internal environment making adjustments and makes endocrine secretions adjust with the sympathetic nervous system. The pituitary gland gets influenced by polypeptide release factors such as CRF from the hypothalamus.

There are many other hypothalamic releasing hormones (RHs) such as growth hormone RH, luteinizing hormone RH, and thyrotropin RH that trigger the release of growth hormones, gonadotropin hormone, luteinizing hormone, and thyrotropin in the anterior pituitary gland. We see the inhibiting action of prolactin and growth hormone by dopamine and hypothalamic somatostatin respectively.

Inhibiting and Enhancing Immune Functions☐

Making electrolytic lesions in the hypothalamus can either inhibit or enhance various immune functions. These changes happen due to the hypophysectomy of the pituitary gland and bring about changes in their function. We can regulate the duration and amount of the immune response. The evidence for this interaction comes from observing specific neurotransmitters, neurohormones, and neuropeptides that influence immune functions. The receptors for the molecules occur on macrophages and lymphocytes.

It is possible to pass on states of arousal to lymphoid tissue through the sympathetic nervous system. The sympathetic nervous system affects both the primary tissues such as the bone marrow and thymus and the secondary tissues such as the lymph nodes and spleen. It is possible to close a negative feedback loop by altering the HPA axis function using cytokines. These cytokines get elaborated from immune cells that get activated.

It is also possible to condition the immune system by pairing a sensory organ with an immunosuppressive drug. When the sensory stimulus is next examined it shows immunosuppressive properties. Many kinds of this bidirectional behavior between the immune system and the CNS exist.

General Adaptation Syndrome Stress Response

Physiological, environmental, and psychological stress can cause distress ("General Adaptation Syndrome: Your Body's Response to Stress", 2020). Activation of the fight-or-flight reaction improves attention span and alertness and it occurs both peripherally and centrally. Together with this, one experiences behavioral adaptation such as aggression and inhibition of vegetative functions such as sexual behavior, feeding, reproduction, and growth.

Peripheral changes include increased heartbeat and blood pressure. We call these changes as General Adaptation Syndrome. There is a redirection of oxygen and nutrients to the organs.

Chapter 19: Have You Heard Of Fibromyalgia?

Considered a complicated health condition, Fibromyalgia affects 1 out of 50 Americans yearly. This condition has no specific cause and still has no known cure. Although the symptoms are treatable and clear -- fatigue, chronic pain and psychological strain, most experts believe that a multifaceted approach combined with medications and changes in lifestyle is the best treatment.

Fibromyalgia: What does it feel like?

Patients with Fibromyalgia experience widespread pain in their muscles. This syndrome however, is caused by other symptoms. Most likely, lab tests cannot validate one's condition and results make a patient feel like a hypochondriac. Whilst you can diagnose Fibromyalgia by pressing on the tender points, this still cannot explain the symptoms.

Likewise, symptoms of Fibromyalgia are often described as a flu-like infection that stays. It leaves the patient exhausted and unable to think and speak clearly which are the symptoms of fibro fog. Moreover, the patient has trouble sleeping and wakes up feeling achy and stiff. The symptoms can be extreme and the patient feels that they are being pushed to get things done.

Several factors influence the cause of Fibromyalgia. Patients of this disease often are discouraged due to the symptoms that are difficult to deal with such as fatigue, sleeplessness and unbearable pain on a daily basis. The confusion surrounding this syndrome, most of the patients are wondering if they are really getting the right diagnosis. Practitioners and specialists are still in the process of seeking answers to the real culprits of Fibromyalgia and also, to find other effective treatments to alleviate its symptoms.

Chapter 20: Looking Forward To The Benefits Of Busting Fatigue

Everyone gets tired. If you've had your fair share of responsibilities, you will most likely have felt fatigued at some point. This does not mean that you should simply yield to what your body is feeling. There are ways through which you can snap out of the rut and boost your vitality. Sure, it can be challenging at first, but you will quickly find that increasing your energy levels for everyday activities all boils down to a few lifestyle tweaks that anyone can successfully pull off. All it really takes is a fair bit of effort and commitment. The fact that you have picked up this book shows that you are at willing to find out about the rest of the process — this actually brings you halfway to your goal already!

Changing your lifestyle to boost your energy levels can provide you with so many benefits for your health, among

A chapter in this book tells you all about what to eat and what not to eat in order to have more energy. Much of the recommended food listed are not just good for making you feel more energetic, but they are also packed with vitamins and minerals that will enable your body to function better. The said chapter will also touch on the recommended portions for the different kinds of food, so you will be able to improve your diet even further.

The process of banishing fatigue also involves doing certain exercises that will strengthen your mind as well as your body. Once you are able to exert the level of commitment necessary to integrate these exercises into your daily routine, you will find it much easier and perhaps even enjoyable to keep being active.

An energetic body and a more organized mind usually go hand in hand. Cultivating the former helps bring about the latter. Changing your diet and becoming more active will keep your mind a lot more awake and open to the possibilities of life around you.

Increased vitality can have you snap out of a rut in more ways than one. As you go along your journey towards better vitality, you may also find that your disposition and perspective on life also improves. After all, it is easier to be more patient and positive about obstacles when your mind, body, and spirit all feel great. The latter can very much be a result of your efforts towards boosting your energy.

Far from simply eating in order to survive, you will learn about the best ways to nourish and fortify your body. Eventually mastering the exercises outlined in one of the succeeding chapters will also endow you with a renewed wonder and awe at what your body is capable of. This new knowledge will then help you become more careful about your lifestyle choices and to take care of your body in a much better way.

Cultivating a healthy lifestyle not only gives you more energy, but it also helps it become stronger. Regular exercise and the right kind of diet will help you build muscles and stamina. Eliminating a few bad habits will allow your body to rest well. As a result, you may find that you are less susceptible to catching the flu or the common cold as compared to before. And who wouldn´t want that?

While the average human being can expect to lose a bit of his vitality every year due to the degenerative effects of aging, that does not mean that there is no way for anyone to boost their flagging energy levels. While doing so would require a considerable amount of effort and commitment, the process is actually quite doable. As the following chapters will show, for individuals who suffer from chronic fatigue, a few small and simple changes in their diet and daily routine can already make a huge difference.

Chapter 21: Internal Stress And How To Deal With It

Internal stress is rooted in our thoughts, opinions, attitudes, beliefs and feelings. Good news is that these are maybe the only things we have direct control over. We cannot change certain situations, our environment or people around us but we can certainly change our attitudes and outlooks. Controlling yourself, of course, is not always easy, but failing to control yourself can end up in you worrying and stressing over absolutely nothing. We generally think that the source of stress is something outside ourselves, but it is actually our internal state that determines whether a certain situation will be stressful for us or not. Once we accept that our internal state is the most, it will much easier to discover ways of coping with internal stress. The range of causes for internal stress is really wide, but we will focus on most common ones.

Do not try to control everything around you

We all sometimes tend to think, and we even try to control everything around us. It is always only a matter of time when we realize that this simply is not possible. This is the point when we start worrying, when we get frustrated, and when the stress arises. So, accepting the fact that basically the only thing we can control and change in this situation is our attitude is the first step in managing this type of stress. Very often some people put a lot of effort in trying to change their partners and failing to do so causes stress. It is possible to guide others, to influence them, inspire and encourage, but it is never possible to control or change somebody, nor should we waste our energy trying. This is the reality of life, and accepting it and staying within our zone of control is a very effective way of coping with stress.

Be aware of your abilities and strengths

To lower internal stress it is really important to know your own abilities and strengths. Setting either too challenging or too small goals can cause stress because we get disappointed either way. However, to learn what you can or what you cannot do depends on your attitude and self-belief. If you set your mind on something, if you put all your efforts and if you firmly believe in your success, even when no one else does, the chances that you will succeed are great. It is important to constantly encourage yourself by positive thinking.

Learn from your mistakes

One more effective way of coping with internal stress is accepting that being wrong or making mistakes is fine as long as you learn something from it. A person who makes mistakes tend to think that they are stupid and worthless, and this way of thinking certainly leads to unnecessary stress. But it should be just the opposite because making mistakes can be beneficial in many ways: it points us to something we did not know, it tells us about our skill levels, it helps us to see what matters and what does not and it encourages us to change something.

Develop your sense of humor

Developing your sense of humor about yourself and your problems does not mean that you do not take your problems seriously. Seeing your troubles in a funny way can cut the level of your stress in half. After all, nothing is bad as it seems.

Build up your self- confidence

Feelings of being unworthy, inadequate or unlovable, i.e. being deeply insecure is one of the biggest causes of stress. When you suffer low self-esteem and when u lack self-confidence, you keep failing in everything you do. The first thing you need to understand is that your pessimistic thinking and your negative attitude brought you there, so you need to change this urgently. You can start getting rid of negative voices in your head by switching to some positive thoughts as soon as you hear negativity in your head. You can also make a list of all your accomplishments and achievements you are proud of. Keep this list always somewhere around you as a constant reminder of how amazing you are. The next thing you can do is to improve your body language. As you appear before others, keep your head up, your shoulders straight, smile more and keep eye contact, because this will firstly make you feel better about yourself and at the same time it will give people impression that you are a confident person.

Chapter 22: Why Do You Need Testosterone?

Whenever you are dealing with the cause and effects of a particular substance, body part or hormone, you are often caught up in a cycle and find it difficult to conclude what actually makes a difference; the cause or the effect. Similarly, researchers run into the problem of determining whether good health ensures optimal levels of testosterone, or whether optimal levels of the same ensure health benefits. However, most findings come up with evidence-led conclusions that show how this hormone plays a number of roles in your life and why you must strive to maintain an optimal level. Listed below are some of the health benefits it contributes to:

It is not unusual to find men struggling to keep depression away, especially in this age of competitive consumerism balancing at the brink of insanity. There is no denying the fact that we have all faced the irritability and instability arising out of the work-life balance, but what is alarming is how the word depression is creeping into the media and our lives as if it's just a regular everyday thing that many people experience on a regular basis.

If you find yourself struggling to stay happy more often than not, you could be suffering from low levels of testosterone. Research suggests that men who have been struggling with symptoms of depression over long periods of time have reported significant improvements in mood after undergoing therapies or treatments to enhance testosterone levels.

It is not easy to deal with everyday troubles that form part and parcel of modern life but it definitely gets easier to deal with life in general when you can identify your ailments and improve your condition. If you have been feeling low or depressed lately, it is time to get in touch with your health practitioner to rule out a deficiency.

Testosterone is known to regulate the fat distribution in the body, keep insulin resistance at bay, and help optimal metabolism of fat. With decreasing levels of testosterone, our bodies struggle to regulate insulin and glucose and with decreasing fat metabolism, adipose tissue begins accumulating.

This is where a vicious cycle takes shape. The increased adipose tissue can to decrease your testosterone levels even further while converting it to estrogen and adding to your troubles.

Needless to say that obese men have lower levels of testosterone and higher levels of estrogen. What is important here is to break the chain of this imbalance and enhance testosterone levels to allow regular distribution of fat.

Men who have undergone testosterone therapies and treatments have reportedly shed weight faster than those relying completely on dietary and lifestyle changes. This is because of the role of this hormone in regulating body fat and insulin glucose.

Have you heard of muscle protein synthesis? Well, that's how testosterone works its way into enhancing muscle mass and strength. If you thought the term 'muscular' was unnecessarily associated with being a man, think again. Have you always envied muscular men taking off their shirt before hitting the showers? Now is the time to put an end to your seemingly miserable life and get your testosterone levels checked. Why? This is because your low level of testosterone may be linked to your diminished strength and low muscle mass.

Conclusion

In summary, fatigue can be caused by one or some causes. Finding the cause of your fatigue is primary in finding the correct treatment to overcome fatigue. Sometimes it is simply too difficult to isolate these causes without professional help. Never consider being tired most of the time 'as normal,' many people are fatigued, but that's doesn't mean it is normal.

There are many possible causes for feeling chronically tired. It's important to rule out medical conditions first, as fatigue often accompanies illness.

However, feeling overly tired may be related to what you eat and drink, how much activity you get or the way you manage stress.

The good news is that making a few lifestyle changes may very well improve your energy levels and overall quality of life.

www.ingramcontent.com/pod-product-compliance
Lightning Source LLC
Chambersburg PA
CBHW071837080526
44589CB00012B/1027